Approaching the
Natural:
A
Health
Manifesto

by
Sid Garza-Hillman
nutritionist/author/philosopher/parent

Library of Congress Control Number:
2012954524

Printed in the United States of America
First Edition
10 9 8 7 6 5 4 3 2 1

Book design by inkfish

Distributed by
Publishers Group West
1700 Fourth Street, Berkeley CA 94710
Phone 510.809.3700
www.pgw.com

Roundtree Press

6 Petaluma Blvd. North, Suite B-6
Petaluma, California 94952
Phone 800.779.5582
www.roundtreepress.com

ISBN: 978-1937359355

To lovely Lisa.

ACKNOWLEDGMENTS

I would like to thank a few folks who played an integral part in helping me write this book. To my patient editor, Stephen Sande, and to Chris Gruener at Cameron/Roundtree Press for getting behind this effort. To Biz Stone for the foreword and for his own good works. To Joan and Jeff Stanford, for providing the venue in which I could launch my nutrition practice. To Jeff Stanford specifically for all the great conversations that helped me hone and refine my approach. To Kim Hillman, brilliant designer and perpetually supportive sister, for making this manifesto look purty. To the great writers Ryan Harty and Julie Orringer for providing encouragement and inspiration. To Scott and Hillary Schneider for taking on additional horse lesson carpooling (long story) that bought me some additional writing time. To Elissa Denker for being a great sounding board and a profoundly courageous person. To Terese Kelley for all her encouragement and ass-kicking. To my wonderful children, Luna, Rónán, and Rinah, for being patient with me during this process, and bravely drinking the "green drinks." And, most of all, to my brilliant, beautiful, and unbelievably tolerant wife, Lisa, for taking a giant leap across the halfway mark of shared responsibilities during the long hours of writing.

contents

Small Is the New Big

My wife and I originally intended to elope in Florence, Italy. When I quit my cushy job to start my own company, we realized Italy was not going to happen. Instead, we discovered the Stanford Inn, a beautiful eco-resort catering to vegans and dog lovers on the Mendocino coast, about three hours' drive from our little place in Berkeley, California. We decided to elope at the Stanford Inn. Jeff Stanford officiated the ceremony himself. It was perfect.

Over the years, we have continued to visit the Stanford Inn at least once or twice annually. On one of our recent trips, a guy named Sid introduced himself while Livia and I were enjoying dinner at the Ravens, the vegan restaurant attached to the Inn. Sid noticed I had ordered a glass of scotch—Laphroig, neat. Suddenly we were discussing peaty scotches with enthusiasm. Sid insisted I try a few of his favorites from what was an extraordinary collection for a vegan restaurant way up in Mendocino.

After a few tastings, I finally got around to asking Sid what his role at the Inn was—assuming he was the sommelier. To my surprise, Sid told me he was the resident nutritionist. Not only that, he was a practicing health coach dedicated to teaching people how to live a natural lifestyle. That's when I realized there was something special about Sid— he wasn't preachy about living a healthy life and that set him apart. Sid's positive and practical approach is his secret weapon.

Far too often, we're told that going vegan or eating healthy means giving up the good stuff. Sid's philosophy turns this around and makes us realize that we're not giving anything up. In fact, the opposite is true—we are gaining something wonderful. A healthy approach to living should be effortless and enjoyable. Unfortunately, this is rarely the way it's presented. Most experts proffer some variation of "no pain, no gain." That phrase is 75% negative. Sid offers us another way—the good way.

Decades of psychology have essentially shown us that positivity works better than negativity. Imagine your dentist asks you, "How often do you floss?" and your answer is, "About two days a week." There are two ways that dentist might react. If she says, "You are a bad patient. I'm disappointed with your lack of diligent flossing," this makes you feel bad. Guess the easiest way to prevent your dentist from saying that to you again? Never go back to the dentist. Your health will most certainly degrade.

Suppose instead that when your dentist asks, "How often do you floss?" your answer remains, "About two days a week," and she responds with, "Great work! Let's try to get that to three or four days a week the next time we meet." You feel good. You're a great patient with the potential to be an even greater patient. Good on you! That positive reaction makes a huge difference. But there's something else going on here—the power of small steps that can take you to your big goals.

When you set a goal like, "Lose fifty pounds," the chances are low that you'll get there. If you do get there, the chances are even lower that you'll stay there. However, if you set a goal of, "No sugary drinks today," then it's almost impossible not to gain momentum. Breaking big goals up into tiny, realistically achievable habits removes will power from the equation. Imagine that. Instead of battling your will power, you are taking tiny steps forward, building momentum, and feeling better every day, every week, every month, and every year. Before you realize it, you're living a natural, healthy, and happy life.

Big goals, broken into tiny habits—even if you fail at them from time to time—will add up to a whole greater to the sum of its parts. In the following pages, Sid will enlighten you. Even this book is little, friendly, and fun. You almost can't help but read it. You'll get to know Sid's affable personality present in these pages. Sid has taught me that approaching a natural lifestyle is a gift, not a struggle. It is my sincere hope that you enjoy this manifesto, and more importantly, enjoy a natural life.

Biz Stone

Co-founder, Twitter

A few years ago I had an idea for a diet book. It was to be about two hundred pages long, and on the cover would be incredible claims like "The diet to end all diets!" and "100% guaranteed weight loss!" Upon opening the book the reader would find the following instructions on the very first page:

1. Eat fruits, vegetables, nuts, seeds, and beans

2. Drink clean water when you are thirsty

3. Exercise every day

The remaining pages would be blank.

Man, what a huge waste of paper that book would have been, and honestly I am probably the only person who finds the idea amusing (that happens a lot). At the same time, after twenty years of studying nutrition, I could not escape a continually nagging suspicion that the subject did not have to be all that complicated. Perhaps it was my philosophy background, but while studying to become a nutritionist I kept asking big picture questions. **1.** Is the human animal really that different from every other animal on Earth when it comes to nutrition? **2.** Do we really need to measure, count, weigh, not to mention process and isolate, what we put in our bodies? **3.** Was there a variety of natural, nutritionally dense foods we could consume and be super healthy without having to rely so much on a bunch of supplements? The more I studied, researched, and learned, the more I became convinced that humans are seriously overthinking the subject of food, nutrition, and health in general.

Once I finished my studies and began my practice, I decided to distill what I had learned into a super accessible and fun format that literally anybody could understand. My intention was to appeal to those who wanted to get healthy, but who were frankly not that interested in the minutiae. I figured that if anyone were as curious as I was about the particulars of human nutrition (the functions of individual vitamins and minerals, digestion, the mechanism of energy creation, molecular biology, biochemistry, and the rest), they would most likely already be reading the same types of books as I.

My classes and consultations continued to evolve, but early on I realized it was simply not enough to provide the information and a plan. Most of my clients would start out strong, but quickly lose steam after the reality of their busy lives took hold once again. I hated the idea that I could be no more effective than a fad diet. In fact, by the time I started my practice I had already seen plenty of friends and acquaintances on "measure this, count that" programs that never lasted, and I did not want to be yet another practitioner doling out unsustainable advice. In the beginning it was both frustrating and disheartening that most of the clients who succeeded in making long-term transitions were those who came to me with already serious health conditions and an immediate, desperate need for nutritional support. I wanted *all* my clients to succeed, no matter their level of health when I began working with them.

Driving home a couple of years ago, I had a bit of an epiphany. There I was, sitting inside a machine that I was controlling with my hands and feet, blocked from the sun, and covered in clothing and shoes. For some reason, driving home in a car, which I had done thousands of times before, seemed utterly crazy in that moment. All of a sudden I became acutely aware that I, like all humans, am an animal— flesh, blood, and bones ultimately made from the earth itself. It was then that the idea for this book came to me. The concept was this: To achieve greater health and happiness, our species need only return by degrees to what is natural to us and in line with our design. It had to do with making choices with an awareness that we were animals so that what was good and not good for us was more obvious. If we behaved less in conflict with our nature, could we achieve greater health and happiness individually and as a species? In other words, could human-inflicted pain and suffering be inversely proportional to how natural we were behaving?

I worked through this idea for a few months and tried applying it to other areas of human life: food, exercise, learning, socializing, creating. It seemed to make sense. Just become more like the thinking human animal you are and your life will improve. But there was one problem: Neither my clients nor I were going to chuck it all and head into the forest to live out our lives. I have a family, a job, a house, a car, places I want to see, and things I still want to do (getting into an airplane and flying to Venice ain't exactly natural, but that is not going to stop me). I had to figure out a way to advocate for a more natural existence while keeping within the framework of the so-called modern world.

So with the basic premise of approaching a more natural state, all I needed was a delivery method that would increase the chances for success. Then it hit me. It was not about going all the way. In fact, what stops many people from beginning the transition to health is their assumption that it would be an enormously huge undertaking and a complete life-change. Most people figure, especially when it comes to nutrition and exercise, that to be healthy they will have to completely turn their lives upside down and give up everything they are used to—buy completely different foods, learn all new recipes, exercise for hours on end, and so on and so forth. I decided it would be more effective to advocate for small steps. And by "small," I mean, well, really small.

I packaged it all up this way: Approach the natural by taking the smallest steps necessary to at least get you to take steps in the first place. In other words, if you don't think you have time for an hour at the gym, try thirty, fifteen, ten, or even five if that will get you going. Better yet, try walking out your door for two minutes, saving the driving time. I thought that if people could just *start* the process, the little steps would eventually become bigger steps. In other words, once they got used to and realized they could manage the two-minute walk, they might try walking for four, or even increasing their speed at some point. Plus, they would begin to feel better along the way (mentally and physically), which is the best motivator.

I began testing my new approach in my nutritional and health coach practice. The results were excellent. I would (and still do) educate my clients first, and then, instead of telling them what they could not or should not do, I would instead say something like this: "If you want to eventually feel better and be healthier, just start for now by adding some of these foods into your daily diet. For now, do not worry about removing anything. Add stuff in, see how you feel, and if you decide to go further, bring in a little more. Eventually you might try decreasing some of the foods you now know are not adding to your health." After a little over a year, with a pile of success stories, I decided to turn my philosophy of health into a book.

The Approaching the Natural philosophy works for a few reasons. First, it is rooted in the knowledge that we are natural beings no matter what we look like and how we act today. As you will read, this simplifies our choices when it comes to health and happiness, especially amidst ever-conflicting studies. Second, the philosophy is gimmick free and long term. It does not yield the immediate highs or subsequent failures that diets, exercise plans, or any other "twenty-one day" type programs do. You ease into it, and therefore have a better chance of sticking with it. Third, the philosophy is about overall health and happiness, and not about specifics like weight loss or a happy marriage. The Approaching the Natural philosophy argues, for example, that healthy weight is merely one side effect of health, just as happy relationships are a side effect of happiness. Finally, the philosophy focuses on the whole human being, and holds that health (body) and happiness (mind) are so intimately related, you need one for the other.

Approaching the Natural: A Health Manifesto was borne out of my own desire to successfully transition my clients to a healthier lifestyle for the rest of their lives—not just with food, but the whole shebang. (What's the whole shebang? Oh, just wait.) I wanted this book to be one that people would keep with them—a book so easy to read, understand, and follow that virtually anyone of any age could immediately start living healthier and happier no matter how busy they were. I wanted it to be, like my classes, accessible and fun, with a bit of humor thrown in, but with absolutely no lists, graphs, or charts. What you are now reading is the end result.

PART ONE

APPROACHING THE NATURAL BODY

chapter one: physical nutrition

When I was a philosophy student, I remember sitting in a class listening to a professor wax philosophic while striking the pose of the thoughtful intellectual gazing out the window, stroking his beard. What he was waxing on about wasn't his own ideas about an ethical dilemma, the nature of the world, or even one of ol' Zeno's paradoxes; instead it was about someone else's ideas and writings (David Hume, in case you're wondering). My point is that much of my studies weren't about philosophy so much as the study of philosophers. Still, my experience in my studies of other's attempts at making sense of the world did get me thinking about things in a much deeper way, and when I later pursued a career as a nutritionist, I couldn't help but ask some bigger questions myself. All this is my way of saying that I'm going to attempt to give you some big-picture thoughts about nutrition and diet in this chapter, and hopefully shed some light on what I think is a mostly unnecessarily complicated subject. Beyond that, my intention is to distill a huge amount of information into a very simple approach, because achieving health is really so much simpler than we are led to believe.

Few subjects are as contentious as nutrition. Unlike animals in the wild, which eat primarily for nutrition and survival —just what they need, no more, no less—the human animal enjoys food in a manner unsurpassed by any other species. Humans reap comfort, security, and sheer pleasure from food, with nutritional concerns often taking a distant second. Early in our lives we learn to associate food with these lovely feelings, and we don't want to give up those tastes or the feelings that are associated with them.

The problem is that many of these foods are not healthy by any stretch of the imagination. Unfortunately, before we are able to make personal choices about what to put in our bodies, we're given foods by our parents, and eventually we latch on to those foods: "Eat your steak, dear." Over time we actually grow to love food we wouldn't naturally be consuming. For instance, one of the big questions I ask is whether our species would naturally be drawn to breast milk from a cow if left to our own instincts and inclinations as children. Ask yourself—when walking by a beautiful pasture full of cows, do you have the urge to get up under one of them and suckle from its teat? Every time you eat yogurt, cheese, or drink a glass of milk, you are in effect doing just that. As children, our parents give us this food (intended for suckling calves) and we grow to love it. The fact that no other mammal on the earth weans from its own mother's milk only to immediately begin breastfeeding from another species certainly raised a few red flags for me. But for most of my clients and students, cheese (which is cow's breast milk, in case you've already intentionally forgotten) is consistently one of the hardest things to give up even though it's one of the least healthy foods a human can consume. Did I just blow your mind? Time after time my clients will hear the facts, and still wrestle with the idea of giving up this supremely unhealthy food. However, the transition to healthy eating is possible, and reading this book will send you on your way.

As a philosopher-nutritionist (kind of like a philosopher-king, but I drive a Ford Focus), it occurs to me that we over-think nutrition to the point of absurdity. We're told carbs are healthy, unhealthy, healthy in moderation, and so on. We're bombarded with information on good fats, bad fats, high-protein, low-protein, and so on and so forth. Then we start counting calories, ounces of water, fat grams, carbs, and everything else under the sun, and to what end? Gorillas in the wild are looking at us like we're insane while they eat the most natural food for their bodies and in amounts that are just what they need. As a species, gorillas are so much healthier than we are that it's not even funny—though I actually think they think it's funny. We are the unhealthiest species on the Earth without exception. So the question is, how is all this nutritional craziness and dieting working for us?

Humans love the idea of quick fixes. We have every diet under the sun available at the click of a mouse, while the most successful of these diets (Atkins, Paleo, etc.) tell us the very foods that give us comfort and security are the foods that will help us shed weight. Half and half in the coffee is good? You betcha. What could be better? The problem is that while these diets can, at best, yield short-term weight loss, they do not deliver long-term health. Diets don't work. We know they don't work, and yet we're always on the lookout for the next diet we think will be the solution to all of our problems.

I get that most people want to eat what they want to eat— namely those foods *that they are used to, that make them feel all that comfort and security.* So what can you do? The simple answer is to stop dieting and begin to move in the direction of health. Learn that you don't have to eat your comfort foods at every single friggin' meal. Then, over time, change what it is that you love to eat—transition yourself to the point where you enjoy healthier foods in the same way you enjoyed unhealthy foods in the past. Yes, it's not only possible, it can happen more quickly than you think. This transitioning is not always easy, however, and I get into that a little later in the book when I delve into ways we can become more mindful in all aspects of our lives. For now, let's consider what the best foods are and how to eat more of them.

*

I'm going to begin with my philosophy of nutrition. Do I think it's the be-all and end-all solution to everyone's problems? No. But I do believe nutrition is the foundation of everything that we are as humans. Give your body the tools it needs to be as healthy as possible and your body will respond, no matter how old you are. The power of feeling good starts with what you put in your body and trickles down to all other aspects of your life—work, relationships, and so on. There's a reason I began this book with a chapter on nutrition...

Because of the sheer amount of food that goes into our bodies, what we eat and don't eat has a profound effect on our lives. We eat more than we do almost anything else in life. In fact, I know people who spend more time eating than sleeping. Many people eat four to six times every day, with additional snacks scattered throughout the day. Make a small daily change to what you do most of the time, and in a year you've affected your body possibly thousands of times.

I have experienced this first hand. In 1992, I had just graduated from UCLA, and was a struggling indie rock musician and long-distance runner with a history of chronic asthma. On my runs I would carry my inhaler with me. Puff before, during, and after a run. That's just the way it was. I come from a family of asthmatics on my dad's side. His mother had asthma, and all his siblings have had it their entire lives. I had some fairly serious asthma attacks as a child. So just genetics, right? As you'll see, there was clearly more to the picture.

Just around that time, a Hollywood actor and his wife, for whom I worked as a personal assistant while a student at UCLA, handed me a book. They were and still are vegan, and I had begun asking them questions. I remember being intrigued, but also in disbelief, that anyone could survive without protein. Naively, I thought at the time that being vegan meant not eating protein. The book they handed me was *Fit for Life* by Harvey and Marilyn Diamond. I read it in a matter of days, and it was a truly life-changing experience. What I thought I knew about nutrition was completely turned on its head. Interestingly, this book was still cited multiple times during my nutrition program in 2009 (published back in 1987, the book still holds up).

The first change I made was to give up dairy—yogurt, cheese, milk, and ingredients such as whey protein powder. My asthma went away almost instantaneously and it has never returned. Similarly, two years ago, my father was able to stop taking chronic asthma medication for the first time in 35 years by following *my* nutritional approach. He is 74 and an avid cyclist. So the "it's just genetics" mantra doesn't always hold water. Give your body the chance to do its job by giving it good food and water, and the return is profound. Our genes are often dispositions rather than the inevitable. They can make us more or less susceptible to environmental influences (like diet), and we can adjust accordingly. Or not. Back in 1992 I could've easily chosen to stick with cheese enchiladas and asthma inhalers. Today, I couldn't be happier that I made the transition to a more natural approach.

*

No matter how brilliantly we are designed—and we are designed brilliantly—if the food we eat is nutrient deficient, our bodies will simply not function well. No yoga, acupuncture, pharmaceutical drugs, or chiropractic care is going to change that. Think of your body as an incredibly well-designed car—mine would be a 1967 Porsche 911. Put dirty oil and gas into the car and it **1)** will not run well; **2)** will eventually break down; and **3)** (most importantly) will not be fun to drive. No matter how much you spend on fancy new tires or a new paint job, if you put dirty oil and gas in the engine, you're going to get the same result every time—an underperforming machine. Humans, as much as we try, do not escape the same fate when it comes to our health. We think we can become healthy by seeing all sorts of health practitioners while still putting bad food in our bodies, but we simply cannot. This speaks to my philosophy of nutrition; namely, nutrition is the foundation of health. The car may need new tires, a new paint job, or might look like all that and a bag of chips with pinstripes running down the side. If the engine isn't running well, don't bother.

In an effort to run the car metaphor to the point of annoyance, even if the engine is running well, you still may need to replace the tires, and throw on some new paint every now and then. Sun, dirty air, and rough roads warrant touch-ups periodically, but a well-functioning engine is essential to drive the car out of the driveway. Get my drift? I promise I'm done with the car thing, but this is precisely why I consider nutrition the foundation and *not* the be-all, end-all solution. We might put the best food possible in our bodies and still need some extra help. Why? Because of the multitude of other ways we are living completely unnaturally.

As a species, humans are so off-the-charts unnatural that most of us need more than good food to make us healthy and happy. We sit for hours in rooms breathing processed air, under fake light, covered in clothing, with chemicals in our hair and on our faces. We are cuckoo. But at the same time, unless we give our bodies the tools to run well, we don't even stand a chance. Being aware of ourselves individually and as a species enables us to make informed, healthy choices. Food is just one of the avenues we can take towards health and happiness. Again, nutrition is not the single solution, but it is the best start. Humans are wading through a world we are simply not designed for, and we need tools to help us. Moving as close as possible to the foods that are most natural to our species is the most powerful tool, but certainly not the only one. In the following chapters, you'll read that in all areas of our lives, the more we simplify, the more we return to our basic needs, the happier and healthier we will be.

The beauty of providing your body with the highest levels of nutrition is that if you still need some outside help (Western medicine, Chinese medicine, Ayurveda), that help will be more effective and able to bring better results. Best-case scenario, I think we can all agree, is that you'll achieve a level of health where you'll rarely if ever need outside help. If I contract a nasty bacterial infection, I'm heading to the nearest MD to get some antibiotics. Just the same, though, I'll do everything I can to *not* get the infection in the first place, dig? Adopting my approach to health has enabled me to stay extremely healthy. I've taken antibiotics one time in the last 12 years. I haven't used an inhaler in 20 years. I don't take Tylenol, aspirin, ibuprofen, Pepto Bismol, or anything like them. That I can live with. Literally. Plug your ears if you're ever told that what you put in your body has no effect on its immune system, because whoever is telling you that is either ignorant or dishonest. Or both.

*

Now we get to the nitty gritty. What do we eat? What is the best diet for us? We are all completely different and need completely different diets, right? Not by a long shot. As you'll see, the very same diet that rocks for diabetes also kicks ass for Alzheimer's, stroke, heart disease, cancer, irritable bowel syndrome, and all those awesome "itis"es like arthritis, bursitis, and my personal favorite, plantar fasciitis (just rolls off the tongue, don't it?).

The differences in nutritional needs from person to person are actually relatively minor, and depend more on the level of stress of the individual than some great biological anomaly. If you're getting four hours of sleep a night, raising a family on your own, struggling financially, and holding down two jobs, your body is going to most likely need more nutritional support than someone who just wants a bit more energy on the golf course, but who is otherwise living a fairly stress-free life. I delve into stress throughout this book, but the long and short of it is that it is supremely difficult to endure chronic stress. After a while that stress will break us down if we're not careful. I'm talking about stress of any kind, by the way, but we add to regular stresses of modern life by eating nutrient-deficient food which creates greater stress to the body and in turn makes it more difficult for the body to endure the life stress—a vicious cycle. The more stress in your life, the healthier you should eat to keep in balance nutritionally.

Here's some basic nutrition 101. All food is made up of macronutrients and micronutrients. Macronutrients are protein, fat, and carbohydrates. Micronutrients are vitamins, minerals, antioxidants, and phytochemicals. By the way, "phytochemicals" just means "plant-chemicals." Man, just turn a word into Latin and you become a fancy-pants. Foods have different amounts and proportions of macro- and micronutrients. The important difference between the two types of nutrients is that macronutrients are caloric. They're all about the energy. Our bodies burn protein, fat, and carbohydrates so that we can move around, think, digest food, eliminate waste, and everything else under the sun. Micronutrients are non-caloric. We need them, but we don't burn them for energy.

Our nutritional problems exist in large part because we are obsessed with macronutrients—protein, fat, and carbohydrates. When you hear "Carbs are bad for me" or "I need to feed my child yogurt to make sure she gets enough protein" or "Coconut oil is bad for me because it's saturated fat," you're hearing statements (all incorrect, incidentally) about calories and energy. In this country the discussion is calorie based, and totally confusing to boot. Remember all that talk about good fats, bad fats, high-protein, low-protein, good carbs, whole carbs, and refined carbs? This kind of talk focuses primarily on energy. If we ever get around to talking about micronutrients—especially vitamins and minerals—it's usually about calcium, iron, and maybe a small handful of others. Don't get me started on why that is. Nice going, you just got me started.

Let me share another personal story. When my wife was pregnant with our twins, she was handed a pregnancy nutrition booklet in her OB/GYN's office. I thumbed through it mostly to distract myself from the "diagrams" on the wall. Besides the fact that the pictures were black and white and looked to be circa 1974, I noticed a few pieces of craziness. One was an entire chart of different meat cuts and the nutritional values of each. The other was a teensy section on vegetarianism that warned that while it was possible to be vegetarian and pregnant, you shouldn't do so without being under the close watch of a health practitioner. The underlying message seemed to be that *not* stuffing yourself with all those delicious saturated-fat-filled flesh cuts was a risky path to take. The kicker was when I read the fine print on the back of the booklet, which stated "Copyright 1988, revised 1992, National Cattleman's Beef Association." By the way, I kept this "pregnancy nutritional guide" and show it to my disbelieving students in all my classes.

Something to keep in mind is that nutritional advice is largely governed by economics, not by health. Evidence is mounting showing the damage high-animal protein diets inflict on our bodies, but there is no counter advertising in the mainstream. The multibillion-dollar food-animal industry currently enjoys a one-sided campaign to keep us buying Big Macs and yogurt. In other words, there is no "Milk, It *Doesn't* Do a Body Good" ad campaign. In my opinion, "Milk, It Does a Body Good" is not objective or well-intentioned nutritional advice. It's an ad campaign, and a darn successful one. This is all fine and good, except that we are becoming unhealthier listening to this crap while continuing to breastfeed from cows. Generation after generation is indoctrinated to believe the human body nutritionally needs two things above all else, protein and calcium. It's simply not true. Period. Let's move on.

Simply stated, for most of us, if we get enough food to eat, we are getting enough calories. Of those calories we consume, some come from protein, some from fat, and some from carbohydrates. Fortunately, in this country most of us do get enough to eat, and yet, again, all we talk about is protein, fat, and carbohydrates—the macronutrients. What is seriously missing from the conversation about food? The micronutrients. We should be asking which micronutrients come packaged with the macronutrients, and in what amounts. In other words, how many different vitamins, minerals, phytochemicals, and antioxidants are hitching a ride with the protein, fat, and carbohydrates in the food we're eating?

We should be asking this because the micronutrients are essential to the proper and efficient functioning of the human body. My apologies for revisiting the car metaphor, but it just works. Eating macronutrients without micronutrients is like putting gas in the car without oil. Gas is the fuel, the macronutrients. A car burns gas for energy just like we burn calories. Oil keeps things clean, efficient, and running smoothly in a well-functioning car. Micronutrients do the same for the body. You've all been behind a car spewing black smoke out the exhaust pipe. The engine is running, but not cleanly. It's suffering from wear and tear. One primary role of vitamins and minerals (micronutrients) is to aid the body in processing the calories. To be healthy we need to create energy in the most efficient and cleanest way possible. When we focus on calories and calories alone and eat foods devoid of micronutrients, we suffer wear and tear. The result is increased waste in the body from energy production, and increased free radical damage. I tackle free radicals and antioxidants in more depth in Chapter Three.

Here's another brilliant metaphor to help simplify food in the hope that you will begin to look at nutrition in a different way. Imagine food as a gift box. The beautiful wrapping on the outside is the calories (macronutrients). Part of that wrapping is protein, part is fat, and part is carbohydrate, but together it's all wrapping. Now let's look at what's inside the gift box. The micronutrients—vitamins, minerals, phytochemicals, and antioxidants. Here's the short story. The heaviness of the box is the determining factor of how healthy the food is: *the heavier the box, the healthier the food.*

By way of example, let's take a gander at the world-famous Big Mac, many of which I consumed as an allergy-laden lad. Let's face it, a Big Mac has gorgeous wrapping—plenty of protein (albeit, an unhealthy form of), carbohydrate (unhealthy form of), and fat (unhealthy form of), but virtually nothing inside the box. The beef (pink slime, anyone?) is primarily protein and fat, as is the cheese. The white flour bun is primarily carbohydrate with a smidge of lab-isolated vitamins and minerals thrown in during the "enriching process." If you're worried about calories, the Big Mac is your ticket, because it's definitely got the calories. But if you're beginning to think about whether or not there's a substantial amount of micronutrients packaged with those calories, then here's your answer. *The Big Mac is a "light box" food.* It's got pretty wrapping, but it's pretty much empty. Compare this to a piece of broccoli, which contains healthy protein (almost 50%, meaning that about half of its "wrapping" is protein vs. about 28% in beef what the? Look it up…), as well as healthy carbohydrate, healthy fat, AND tons of stuff inside the box. *Broccoli is a "heavy box" food.* More bang for your buck, and a whole host of other clichés. What you get with the kick-ass broccoli is the heaviness of vitamins, minerals, antioxidants, and phytochemicals, all mixed up with fiber that helps the nutrients end up where they are supposed to go. For the record, you also get plenty of protein, fat, and carbohydrate when you eat your broccoli. Basically, the more "heavy box" foods you include in your life (a variety of whole fruits, vegetables, seeds, and nuts), the healthier you're gonna be. These are foods the body can process cleanly, efficiently, and with minimal stress. For the record, chimpanzees in the wild eat 100% "heavy box" foods that are designed to work with the body. Gorillas thrive primarily on whole plants. They seem to be getting enough protein, don't you think?

Now we're getting into the heart of this here piece o' literature. For a species that is the self-proclaimed most intelligent on the planet, you would think we'd have done a tad bit better with our health. Instead, we seem to think, in all our arrogance, that we are smarter than Mother Nature. We find resveratrol in a grape and discover it has incredible health benefits. But instead of eating the grape, which is a "heavy box" food, we extract the resveratrol and stick it in a pill with fillers and such. Genius. How's that working for us? Are we healthier, and how are we feeling day to day? Natural food, food from the earth (like the grape), has it all: macronutrients and micronutrients in exactly the right way and in the right amounts for that food. Eat a wide variety of these foods and you'll give your body everything it needs. Just put it in there and let your body suss it out.

Nutrients neither exist in isolation nor function in isolation. We can't recreate health in a pill. When I was studying to become a nutritionist I had to memorize the list of nutrients, and for each one, there was an adjunct list of the other nutrients it needed to do its job. Guess which nutrients we need? The answer is all of them. Of course we need protein, but we also need carbohydrates and fat, and we need healthy versions of all three. Of course we need calcium, but we also need iron, magnesium, copper, zinc, phosphorous, potassium, and more. When you get these nutrients from food rather than pills you're going to achieve better health. The idea is to eat a variety of heavy box foods, mostly raw and whole plants. Do that and you got it going on. With the exception of vitamin D and B12, my family and I get all our micronutrients from food, and we have never been healthier. Furthermore, we do not take vitamin D when we get enough sun, and only take B12 because we wash the plants we eat (B12 is produced in our bodies from microorganisms found in soil).

Here's what happens when we focus on one nutrient. The United States hovers at the top of the list for calcium consumption, yet we suffer from some of the worst bone health in the world. One explanation for this is that our bones aren't just made of calcium. Bones contain phosphorus, magnesium, zinc, boron, and other minerals, while vitamin D regulates the absorption of calcium into the bones. In addition, acid-forming foods in our diet force the body to take calcium from the bones. Calcium is an alkaline mineral, and the body uses it to buffer/neutralize any increasing acidity in blood. Once used in the blood, calcium ends up leaving our bodies through our urine. As Dr. Joel Fuhrman describes it in *Eat to Live*, "Epidemiologic studies have linked osteoporosis not to low calcium intake but to various nutritional factors that cause excessive calcium loss in the urine. The continual depletion of our calcium reserves over time, from excessive calcium excretion in the urine, is the primary cause of osteoporosis." He then lists dietary factors, including animal protein, salt, caffeine, and refined sugar that result in a loss of calcium. Yet most health practitioners advise us to consume more calcium for improved bone health, instead of showing us how to prevent the loss of this mineral.

Here's the 411. Foods we eat can affect the acid/alkaline balance of our blood. Our blood sits in the slightly alkaline realm: pH of 7.4 to 7.5. pH is potential of hydrogen, and I mention that only so that you think I'm pretty great.

When we eat food, there is a post-digestion residual or ash that can move the body to more acidity or alkalinity depending on the nature of the food. Understand this point: it is not about the acidity of the food itself, but the pH of the ash/residue. Lemons are acidic tasting, but alkaline-forming in the body, got it? Also, there is some misinformation about the acid/alkaline balance (big surprise). It's not that your body can become super acidic if you consume acid-forming foods. If your blood becomes super acidic, you'll die, sorry to say. The concern is how much work you are creating for your body to maintain its proper pH. As I stated above, the body's solution to increased acid load involves a series of reactions resulting in calcium being depleted from the bones in an effort to neutralize the increasing acidity. The amount of acid-forming foods you consume directly affects the acid/alkaline balance in your body.

As a nutritionist, I focus on minimizing intake of acid-forming foods, because the typical modern diet is mostly made up of them, and we're suffering for it. Add to that the fact that stress, fear, anger, and anxiety also increase body acidity and it becomes super important to tip the scales in favor of alkaline foods. As you'll read in chapter 4, chronic stress of any kind, nutritional, emotional or otherwise, takes a heavy toll on the body, including weakening the immune system. Bad news for health and happiness. With my clients, most of my work involves helping to introduce more and more alkaline-forming foods into the diet, with the idea of minimizing nutritional stress on the body.

So which foods are typically acid-forming, and which are alkaline-forming? Hopefully this isn't a shocker, but "light box" foods increase the acid load on the body, while "heavy box" foods high in micronutrients increase the alkaline load. "Light box" foods like refined white flours, white rice, animal protein, dairy and soy protein isolate, plus prescription drugs and synthetic vitamins, are all highly acid-forming. These are the things we consume that the body just doesn't recognize. They also require a huge amount of work to deal with. "Heavy box" foods like whole fruits, vegetables, seaweed, and seeds are alkaline and chock full of micronutrients our bodies need. Flood your body with "heavy box" foods and you make it easier for your body to stay in balance. Less work means less stress on the body. Follow this thinking and you don't need to worry about acid, alkaline, counting calories, protein grams, calcium milligrams, or whatever other craziness we humans take on.

So how did I come to the conclusion that a mostly raw, whole plant diet is the most natural to humans? Good question, because we all know that meat-eating is part of the history of our species. But it's just not that simple. I do not deny, and have never seen evidence to contradict the fact that humans have always eaten meat. I hear this all the time in my classes, and currently, the Paleo diet is the hot new diet everyone's talking about. The gist of the Paleo diet is that we should eat the food our ancestors ate between 10,000 and 2.5 million years ago: pre-dairy, pre-processed food, pre-added salt and the like. For the record, not all bad advice in my opinion, except the Paleo diet weighs too heavy on flesh eating. Many people use the Paleo diet as an excuse to eat meat all the time, just like they did with Atkins. But diets like these fail to recognize some very significant differences between meat-eating of today and that of yesteryear, and by the way I just took pleasure in being able to use yesteryear in a sentence.

First of all, just because humans *can* digest flesh doesn't mean that it is optimal for health. While there is conflicting evidence regarding the amount of flesh consumed by our species historically—some claim as low as 5% of our calories came from flesh—no one is disputing the fact that we also consumed whole plants. Interestingly, in his book *Born to Run*, Christopher McDougall writes that meat-eating was most likely out of need of a calorie boost. If experiencing a deficit of edible plant foods, our ancestors would kill an animal to get what they needed for energy. In this day and age, and especially in this country, micronutrient and calorically dense plants (i.e. nuts and seeds) are super easy to come by, rendering flesh-eating virtually unnecessary. Secondly, the meat many of us are eating today is substantially different from the meat we ate during the Paleolithic period. For this let me verbally paint you a picture.

Imagine a fairly hairy, upright-walking gentleman strolling (and probably running, as you'll see in the next chapter) through the forest looking for food. Once in a while that food would be a wild animal. This animal was running around and trying to not be killed by our distant ancestor, whom we'll call Uncle Thak. So what about it? The prey Uncle Thak hunted differed from the animals we eat today for several reasons. **1)** This animal was running around in the wild, and all that exercise resulted in leaner flesh. **2)** This animal was eating wild plants grown in nutrient-rich soils (or eating another animal that was eating the plants). **3)** This animal was drinking clean, natural, hydrating water. **4)** Our Uncle Thak ate his meat raw and fresh unless he had a dorm fridge and hot plate. And lastly, **5)** Thak wasn't eating meat every meal or even every day—again, probably only when he was facing a caloric deficiency. Thak, therefore, is the very picture of a person (albeit a very hairy person) who is seriously "Approaching the Natural."

Unfortunately, in the modern world, we are consuming very different animals. **1)** The animals we eat are kept in a confined space, have no need to exercise as they're not in danger from natural predators, and don't need to search for food. This allows them to get nice and fat. **2)** We're feeding our animals cultivated plants grown in overplanted soils, many subjected to herbicides and pesticides, AND on top of that often feeding them food that is completely unnatural to them. For example, most cows are fed corn, soy, and all sorts of other non-cow food (they are naturally herbivores and should be eating grass). In addition, cows are pumped full of hormones, antibiotics, and whatever else we human f'n geniuses can think of. **3)** These herded animals are drinking water full of chemicals and toxins, the list of which is truly frightening, and which are mostly stored in the animals' fat that people are slurping down. **4)** Most meat-eaters ain't eatin' steak tartar if you catch my drift, and who knows how old the rotting muscle is by the time it hits the super hot grill/pan/flame and then the table. And lastly, **5)** Most Americans are eating flesh, or some sort of animal food, at nearly every meal. This is so far from "Approaching the Natural" that we're living in Cuckoo Town (just east of Tulsa).

Just because our species has a history of doing something does not necessarily mean it is natural to us. In fact, many horrible things we have historically done, I would argue, are a result of our species acting in conflict with our design. We have a history of murder, genocide, racism, and sexism, all of which ain't exactly making humans the heroes of the Earth. Regardless of what we have done in the past, we can look at the makeup of the human body, the physical attributes, and draw a pretty easy conclusion that all things being equal, our bodies thrive on whole plants. Yes we can survive on a whole host of other foods—the muscle, organs, breast milk of animals, and Twinkies for that matter—but what foods will make us the healthiest and happiest? We are able to stay alive eating Big Macs, but do we *feel* alive doing it? The comparatively long length of our intestines, our opposable thumbs, our ability to move our jaws side to side, teeth that are perfect for peeling and grinding, our only moderately acidic environment stomachs (compared to the highly acidic stomachs of carnivores and omnivores), and a carbohydrate-digesting enzyme in our saliva (amylase) allows for the efficient processing of plants.

If I were living on a tundra, (and please someone tell me what the hell a tundra is), I'd most likely hunt and kill animals to survive. I still wouldn't suckle on 'em, though. Why? Because I'd lack access to enough plants to satisfy my energy needs. I would require a fuel source to produce the amount of energy needed for survival, and I'd find the best quality source possible. I live in a fairly remote small town on the Mendocino Coast of Northern California (real northern, not San Francisco). Still, the closest thing to hunting in my town is finding the prettiest tomato of the bunch at the organic market seven minutes from my house. The cleanest, healthiest energy source is always within reach because I have easy access to a huge variety of heavy box foods including fresh fruits, vegetables, seeds, and nuts.

The research I've done for the last 20 years has led me to conclude that all this is really quite simple. I don't count calories, fat grams, or carbs (least favorite abbreviation by the way—THANKS, Dr. Atkins!); I don't check which foods are high on the glycemic index; I don't make sure my meals are "balanced" or anything else of that sort. What I figured out a long time ago is that the human body is way more intelligent than the human mind. Give your body the tools it needs to be healthy and your body will make it happen. But how do you get there? What are the nuts and bolts of transitioning yourself to a better diet? "I'm begging you for the info, Sid. Give it to me straight," I'd be glad to.

Most humans are far from "natural." The farther away you are, the less healthy you are going to be. In your quest to be healthy and happy, start to move closer to our species' most natural state and the healthier and happier you will be. All you need to know is what the most natural state looks like; the closer you get, the better. So let's see how Approaching the Natural can apply to food.

Let's start with the chicken-fried steak served for lunch at my high school. Loved it: the chicken-fried steak, not the high school. Let's say you eat that chicken-fried steak or something comparable on a daily basis, and that your cholesterol and blood pressure are as high as your belly is round. You may be asking why this "fictional you" would still eat this crap? Maybe it's because so-called "dieticians"are still recommending high-protein diets. To sound healthy they will advise white meat, skinless chicken, and low-fat dairy. They're like broken friggin' records. Light boxes, my friends, but I digress. For the sake of this little exercise, let's just say you agree with the premise that what you put in your body affects your health…you know, 'cuz it does.

So in your high-cholesterol, high-blood-pressure, heavy-belly hypothetical life you decide it's time to make a change, but you aren't ready to go "all granola." Here's what you do—"Approach the Natural." Take a first step. This might be switching from chicken-fried steak to a broiled chicken. Hang out there for a while. Another move, you say? How about the skinless white-meat chicken all the kids are talking about? Hmmm. Not much change? How about going to a grilled tofu on top of that Chinese chicken salad instead of the chicken? After that try replacing the tofu with some cashew cheese for a while, then moving on to some raw cashews and hemp seeds, and so on and so forth until you reach what I believe is the most natural diet for humans. I'm talking about raw, whole plants plain and simple: *fruits, vegetables, nuts, and seeds of all different colors, shapes, and sizes.*

The point is that you don't have to go from chicken-fried steak to raw plants in one move. Of course you can if you want, but for that matter, you don't have to move at all—you're just not going to get healthy if you don't. My goal is to make you super aware of the very well-researched fact that what you eat is the most profound determining factor of your overall state of health, and that if your current state of health is not to your liking, to teach you how to change it. Period. Just as a point of reference, I don't even hit the natural all the way. But I'm darn close, and if I'm feeling fatigued, achy, or anything other than dandy, guess where I go? I go to the natural. But I love my single-malt Scotch and I love my home-roasted espresso beans. I don't overdo either (Scotch maybe once a month, can't say the same for coffee…), and I'm as healthy as I want to be. If at some point I'm not, I'll know exactly what to do and where to go (one thing being to give up the single-malt Scotch and coffee...oh the horror). Approaching the Natural is about minimizing light box foods and maximizing heavy box foods by degrees. The more you tip the scales in favor of heavy boxes, the better you'll feel.

*

A lot of my nutritional practice involves reminding people to keep their eye on the ball. The goal is simply to be and feel healthy. Weight loss, for example, is simply one side effect among many that comes with a healthy body. If my goal as a nutritionist were weight loss, I'd throw everyone on the Atkins Diet, or a whole host of other crazy short-term fixes. I'd collect my dough and be a hero for six months. But I wouldn't be able to sleep at night knowing I recommended foods that were at best unhealthy, and at worst, dangerous.

I still have clients who listen to my recommendations and then proclaim that it's just impossible for them to give up cheese, to which I respond, la di da. Man, they love that response. But I go on to say this: If you want to be healthier, "Approach the Natural." If you want to be the healthiest you can be, go all the way. If you're fine with your current level of health, don't change a thing. It's not too complicated when you think about it. If you love cheese more than you love being healthy, more power to you. There are other considerations, and bigger pictures involved, which I'll delve into later in the book.

*

So to my bearded professor of yesteryear, thanks for the memories. My hope is that by de-mystifying nutrition and diet, and then by showing you the clear picture of the very healthiest diet, you at least know where to go if you want to. I can't stress enough that it's up to you at the end of the day. Nobody is, or should be, telling you what to do. My hope is that you "Approach the Natural" because YOU choose to.

In the next chapter I'll apply my philosophy (shazam!) to the movement of our bodies. I begin this book with a chapter about food because, as I've mentioned, this is where it all starts. Get the ball rolling toward the healthiest diet ever, and you'll be better equipped to pursue whatever it is you want to do. But moving our bodies, you know, getting off the couch, is also crucial to our health and happiness. As you'll see, just as it is with food, even taking the smallest step can have a profound effect on your quality of life.

chapter two: moving

Good health, and the happiness that comes with feeling and being truly healthy, is not complete without considering the whole picture of the human experience. The previous chapter addressed what we put in our bodies. This chapter deals with what we *do* with our bodies. I'm talking about moving.

When discussing movement—exercise, working outside, getting jiggy wid it, or whatever you choose to call moving your body—it is easy to agree that "Exercise is good for you," just as it's easy to conclude that "Eating healthy is good for you." But knowing what constitutes healthy food and healthy movement is a different matter altogether, not to mention the struggle that comes with figuring out how to incorporate healthy eating and movement into your life. The conventional wisdom surrounding health is generally not healthy at all, and in fact can get us into trouble. This book is about exploring the layers of knowledge that lie underneath the conventional wisdom.

When it comes to health, what most people normally do to be healthy is rarely beneficial. In fact, "normal" has become only what most people do, rather than a statement about what is most in line with our nature and design. For instance, drinking cow's milk is seen as normal, acceptable, and supremely healthy, and those who don't indulge are labeled weird or somehow abnormal. We've all heard from an early age how cow's milk is essential for human beings. This is conventional wisdom at its finest, and dietitians across the country are still recommending milk as if they couldn't stop themselves if they tried. Likewise, much that comprises our lives—cell phones, cars, fast food, air conditioning, and such—is "normal" by society's standards but quite odd when you consider that we are, at the end of the day, animals on a planet. So in the realm of movement, just because most people hardly move their bodies doesn't mean it is natural or normal. It is typical but not normal. Unfortunately, the most natural things for us to do are often perceived as crazy.

*

Regarding natural human movement, there are two different issues as I see it: **1.** *whether we're moving enough* and **2.** *how we are moving.* To tackle number 1, let's look at what is clearly not natural. Take a gander at what might be a typical day for some of you or people you know…

> You wake up in the morning, grab your coffee (roasty goodness), and you're in the bathroom getting ready for work. Into the kitchen you go for a bowl of cereal and milk, fried eggs or yogurt (conventional wisdom: all you need is protein and calcium) and head out the door. You get in your car and drive thirty minutes to the office where you park, get out of the car, enter the building, get into an elevator, and exit at your floor. Once in your office or cubicle, you take a seat at your desk in front of the computer and work away for a few hours. You take a lunch break either at your desk or sitting in a restaurant somewhere close by. At the end of the day you take the elevator back down to the parking lot and get back into your car. You make the thirty-minute drive home, perhaps stopping for drive-thru eats on the way. You park

in your driveway, enter, and sit in front of a television or computer screen and watch a movie in your comfy la-Z-Boy chair that may or may not have a cooler built into the armrest. When you finally get tired, you head into the bathroom, brush your teeth (don't forget to floss), climb into bed, and it's lights out.

Think about this for a minute. A lot happened during your day—activity, productivity, and even entertainment. But what's missing? The short answer is *movement*. In that whole day of busy stuff and fun, there was a substantial *lack of any movement*. The totality of exercise amounts to short walks at best—house to car, car to office, office to lunch, lunch to office, office to car, car to home. The question we need to ask is how this meshes with the design of our species. Is this type of day-to-day living natural? While we can't disregard the logistical necessities of modern living (i.e. working in offices, driving in cars, etc.), in the context of the millions of years of our evolution, the answer is clearly no.

In our ultra-modern world, we presently have the unique distinction of achieving almost 100% stagnation due in large part to technologies that enable us to get things done with little physical effort. Cars, e-mail, cell phones, tractors, you name it. We can do much of the business of our lives from a table at Starbuck's. We can order groceries, talk to our friends, and transfer money from checking to savings (or vice versa, as my case may be). To send a message, we don't even have to get up and grab a stamp or an envelope. These days it's just click and send. But we're paying a heavy price (way more than the cost of a stamp) for sitting on our butts most of the time. In the not-to-distant past, Pa and Half-pint had to engage in a lot of activity and travel quite the distance from that little darn house on the prairie just to send a letter (and that was just across a Hollywood studio lot).

Our species has distanced itself from movement. Once we moved out of necessity: gathering, hunting, building, relocating etc. It was an integral part of our lives—don't move and you die. Actually the same thing applies to human beings today, but it is subtler than that. The idea of moving just for the benefit of moving is relatively new and completely unique to us. Back in the proverbial day, we didn't go to a prehistoric gym (the rock-climbing walls were authentic back then, I can tell you), beat the crap out of our bodies for 35 minutes, hustle back to work red-faced and sweaty before our bosses got annoyed, and all of a sudden become known as the "always sweaty red-faced guy" around the office.

Instead of exercise being integrated into the activities we need to perform each day, it is now an add-on to our lives. We have a list of things to do, and exercise is one of them. I get it. I'm there too. I'm not on a mini-tramp every morning because jumping up and down in my living room is what it takes to gather blackberries from the bushes along my driveway. I'm a modern animal busy with the tasks of living in a modern world, so to move my body I have to carve out time for a condensed and intense workout. By the way, I do manage to pull this off with three-year-old twins so, you know, I'm busier and more tired than you are, so quit your complaining. But the reality of my life is anything but atypical. While some professions are physical in and of themselves, most humans in the modern world have to make an effort to include any movement whatsoever in their lives.

*

If a typical modern day's worth of activity is severely lacking in movement, what should the goal be? Just how much should we all move? There's no simple answer because there's no fixed "right" amount that applies to everyone, just as eight cups of water per day isn't the "right" amount for every single person no matter their height and weight (oh, the things we are nutty nut nut about…). However, for every person there is both too little and too much movement. The trick is finding the right balance.

Part of finding the right balance of movement means taking nutrition into account, as the two are intimately related. Each substantially affects the other in the context of health. In Chapter One I wrote about the benefits of heavy box foods. Adding movement into the picture, health becomes not only about the quality of food you eat, but also the quantity of food for the movement (work or exercise) that your body performs each day. Moving too much or too little in relation to the amount of calories you've consumed adds stress to your body. Moving around in the right way and in the right amount can give you the well-established and amazing benefits of exercise. Too little or too much movement and your body suffers. It is essential to make sure you have the right amount of nutrients and calories so that your body has the support it needs to handle the level of activity. For example, athletes, farmers, and accountants all need heavy box foods to be healthy, but each might need to consume more or less calories than the others depending on the amount of physical work he or she performs each day. When there is imbalance, there is stress.

I write about stress throughout this book because stress is a biggy in my nutritional practice. Pretty much the biggest for me ("biggiest"—yes it's a word…as of right now) because chronic stress wreaks havoc on our bodies. As a nutritionist I try to provide an appropriate level of nutritional support for the amount of stress they are under. Why? Because, as I wrote in the previous chapter, one effect of chronic stress is that it weakens the immune system. Bruce McEwen, in *The End of Stress as We Know It*, explains the difference between short-term stress and long-term stress: "Under acute stress, the immune response is enhanced. The infection-fighting white blood cells attach themselves to the blood vessel walls, ready to depart for whatever part of the body is injured. But if a stressful situation goes on too long, the immune response is dampened in favor of the primary systems—the heart and lungs—that need the energy most" (p. 6). The body's stress responses are designed for the short term, and all are focused on one thing and one thing only: survival. Too much or too little movement in our lives can contribute to chronic stress, and the effects on the body are truly fascinating and awe-inspiring in an odd sort of way. Kind of the way that I'm still blown away by technology that Gen Y'ers take for granted. Seriously, Google, how do you do it?

Another effect of chronic stress is that it increases fat around the midsection, and makes it easy for us to put on, and keep on, extra fat. Again, Bruce McEwen writes, "Too much cortisol [a hormone, increased levels of which occur during stress] blocks the actions of insulin to stimulate muscle to take up glucose. An excess also enhances the storage of energy in an unsightly manner—fat, particularly abdominal fat, which is thought to pose more of a health threat than fat around the thighs and hips. Cortisol promotes the loss of protein from muscle and converts it to fat…" (p. 24). Using this paradigm, it becomes possible to assess the amount of stress on an individual just by checking out their waistline. If there's a big ol' gut hanging over your belt, chances are your body is under some serious stress, which could be from a whole host of things including too little or too much exercise, too much exposure to the jackass in the next cubicle, or a diet made up of light box foods — that muffin top around your middle could be from eating too many muffin tops. My point is, the body will exhibit a stress response no matter the source of the stress.

Yet, in spite of the debilitating effects of chronic stress, the human body still manages to stay alive and be productive. It is amazing that people can treat their bodies so poorly and still get up in the morning and negotiate the world, much less run a half marathon. In fact, while running half marathons I've been passed by people who are substantially overweight. I've also seen plenty of people who work out like banshees at the gym and just can't seem to lose the extra weight. Even though these folks are able to perform these activities, I see them as suffering from stress. The problem is that because they can still pretty much function day-to-day, they just keep doing the same exercise regimen or diet, hoping that all of a sudden they'll hit a healthy weight. What they most likely need to do is either improve the quality and quantity of their nutrition, or dial back the intensity of their exercise. Either way, what's clear is that there is an imbalance. Of course, if you asked one of these people how it is that they can exercise so much and not be at a healthy weight, you'd probably hear a few familiar excuses. The most common are age and genetics: "This is just what happens when you get older," "I'm just built this way," or "It's genetics." I understand the relief that comes from believing that achieving health is out of our control, but the truth is that most often it is very much in our control.

Instead of trying to combat excess fat with dieting, extreme exercise, drugs, or crazy amounts of costly supplements and protein powders, a healthier course of action would be to find ways to remove or minimize stress so your body can do what it's constantly trying to do, which is to be as healthy as possible. Brendan Brazier, a professional ultra marathoner, triathlete, and author of *Thrive Fitness* puts it this way: "After overconsumption, the greatest reason for obesity in North America is that we are simply inundated with more stress that we can deal within a sustainable, healthy manner." He writes about those people who exercise a bunch but just can't lose the excess weight: "Despite consistent exercise, they can't lose extra body fat or reshape their body…the underlying problem may be too much stress—from several sources—which culminates in a variety of health problems" (Pg. 52). Brazier actually recommends stopping exercise for a while. He suggests taking some time off to allow the body to normalize a bit, before beginning again with a more appropriate and balanced level of exercise.

It is true that exercise itself can help relieve stress, but only when performed in a balanced way. Going for a long walk or a comfortably paced run feels incredible and can relieve the stress of the day. A jump on my rebounder works for me when I need to burn off some excess energy—mental or physical (kind of like a Manhattan up, but a bit healthier). A punching bag does wonders to burn off some anger, trust me. Balanced exercise can help dissipate stress without adding stress.

*

So, if you want to know how to get your butt moving again, read on. The goal is to re-incorporate movement and return to a state much closer to our nature. I'll first explore movements that are most natural to our species, because even when we're exercising in the right amount, and with the right quality and quantity of our food, there are certain movements that minimize the risks of injury and stress to our bodies. These movements might be just the place to start when making the choice to "Approach the Natural." After that I'll show you steps you can take to actually get moving again in a sustainable way that minimizes the chances of burnout.

So what movements are most natural to humans? Walking surely comes to mind, and recent research suggests that running is a big part of the picture, as well. Makes sense, right? We walk, we run. Both have been our main mode of getting around, and even relatively stagnant humans walk to get from the bed to the bathroom or the kitchen to the car. If you're late for the bus, you're going to run to catch it.

Human beings are also super-efficient long-distance runners. In fact we may be the best long-distance runners on the planet, because of the way our bodies are designed. Christopher MacDougal's book *Born to Run* set off a movement (no pun intended) to return to our roots as running animals, and he makes a convincing case that humans evolved to be natural runners. Our tendon-filled bodies allow us to be springy. Our relatively hairless bodies and our ability to sweat allow us to keep fairly cool while we run. Our upright, bipedal gait (walking vertically on two feet) minimizes the surface area of the body that is exposed to direct sunlight. Combined, these attributes enable humans to run long distances in a very efficient manner with minimal stress. In short, we were built to run.

Many people respond to the thought of running with concern that it leads to injuries. Indeed, I've met plenty of "former" runners who have given up running because their knees, hips, or backs gave out and who are now biking or swimming. The potential for injury definitely keeps many people from running in the first place. So, if running is supposedly natural for us, why are there injuries? The answer is that running is natural when (and this is a big "when") we run in the *style that is most natural to our bodies*. We suffer injuries because we no longer run the way we were designed to.

In order to explain, consider our feet. If you wear shoes, especially running shoes, take a gander at them. Basically, we have taken two incredibly brilliant and intricate pieces of machinery—the feet, which are designed to support our entire weight and are filled with more nerve endings than almost anywhere else on our bodies—and we've covered them with rubber, leather, mesh, padding, and laces. We've smothered, trapped, constrained, babied, padded, and confined them. The feet ain't out in the world free to do their thing, and it's a problem.

We force our feet into laziness when we constrain them in shoes. The information the feet are designed to provide us is completely cut off by the thick soles of shoes. We are instinctually drawn to read and negotiate the ground with our feet, and simply can't when we separate them from the surface on which we're walking. Padded shoes block essential environmental feedback including rough terrain, bumps, holes, and dips. In fact, runners in padded shoes actually strike the ground harder than barefoot runners. It is as if the foot is trying desperately to feel what's underneath it but can't. Unfortunately, the harder the foot strikes the ground, the greater the bodily impact, which in turn means increased chance of injury. Statistics show that the most injuries suffered by runners are overwhelmingly from those wearing shoes. Again, in our effort to outsmart Mother Nature, we pay a heavy price. Now let's take a look at what we did before we decided that Mother Nature couldn't do for us what Zips running shoes could.

In short, up until very recently in our evolution, we ran either barefoot or with virtually no padding or arch support on our feet (e.g. moccasins or sandals). Running barefoot is more natural and less stressful on our bodies. When we run in the barefoot style we actually run in a completely different way. We return, you guessed it, to the gait most natural to our species—running lightly on the balls of our feet that softly land right beneath our hips, and with slightly bent, bouncy legs. No straight leg heel strikes, no jarring impact on our knees, hips, and back, even when running on concrete. I've been running barefoot either completely, or in my Vibram five fingers, for three years now and I'll never go back.

In the interest of full disclosure and to hopefully prevent you from doing what I did, I injured myself when I first began running barefoot, but not because it is an unnatural way to run. Here's how it happened. When I first got my Vibrams I went for a couple short runs and it felt so dang good that I ran an eight miler. Lo and behold, I stress-fractured my foot. Why? Because I hadn't taken the time to develop the muscles in my feet that had for so long been severely under-used. In other words, I didn't "Approach" anything. I just rushed all the way in and my feet couldn't handle it. It was like I walked into a weight room for the first time and attempted a 250 lb. deadlift—not a pretty picture.

My injury was such a letdown, because those first barefoot runs were the most exhilarating of my life. I learned my lesson, however. After recovering, I read *Barefoot Running* by Michael Sandler (more on learning in Chapter Four) and took the necessary time to build up the muscles in my feet through special foot-strengthening exercises and by running very short distances. I increased the distance incrementally over about a year's time. I would run a tenth of a mile barefoot for about a week and then increase it by another tenth the following week and so on. It took a while, but now I can run in the barefoot style any distance I want (or, more accurately, can). It feels absolutely incredible. I get asked about my shoes all the time, and I sound like a religious convert when I tell people how great it feels to use my feet again. But it does. Anyone who knows me will attest to the fact that when running or not, I'm either completely barefoot or in Vibrams almost 100% of the time. I've got a work pair and a running pair, though I probably shouldn't have admitted that.

Not only is the barefoot style of running more in line with our physical design, running on natural ground takes the cake too. Just consider the difference between running on a treadmill versus a road versus a trail. The treadmill is a perfectly flat and very controlled surface. Roads, while being a little more imperfect (or perfect depending on how you look at it), are still a far cry from truly natural terrain. Natural ground like trails offer ups, downs, and side-to-sides, and little breaks in between. How does this benefit us?

Running on natural terrain delivers a whole body exercise. Essentially it is interval training the natural way—moving with varying intensity levels and heart rates (i.e. running as fast as you can for a minute, then walking or lightly jogging for a minute, or even running up and down hills). The benefits of this type of exercise are well established. Interval training promotes lean muscle growth and fat loss, triggers the release of human growth hormone, and strengthens the heart. Michael Fossel, Greta Blackburn, and Dave Woynarowski, in *Immortality Edge*, write that interval training "leads to an adaptive response. The body begins to build new capillaries, and it is better able to take in and deliver oxygen to the muscles. The muscles, in turn, develop a higher tolerance to the buildup of lactate, and the heart muscle is strengthened" (Pg. 86-87). Running with a natural gait in natural terrain provides a varying heart rate because you have to negotiate turns, hills, soft ground, hard ground, logs, and everything else. Also, running outside on natural earth is about as good as it gets because of the added benefit of the sunlight, fresh air, and surrounding beauty. It's almost otherworldly except that really it couldn't get more "worldly." Unfortunately we have become a society where running inside on a rotating belt is somehow more normal than running barefoot through a forest.

*

No matter who you are, it's important to move. Let's face the facts: We're not built physically or psychologically to live stagnant lives and we exist in a state of conflict when we do. Using my "our body as a car" analogy from before, if you don't drive your car, the engine will eventually suffer damage from sitting for too long. Stop moving the machine and it wastes away over time. Same thing happens to our bodies. We're like rusting cars on the front lawns of life... wow, did I just write that? Where's the damn delete key?

I'll get into the particulars of the first steps we can take below, but the idea is simple: moving is better than not moving. Obviously I love walking and running, but if you dig your spin class, have at it. If Bikram yoga floats your boat, Bikram up—though doing anything other than lying down in a room heated to 105 is just ridiculous. OK, I admit that is not fair. It's just that I don't do well in heat and have never actually taken a Bikram yoga class. Plus it's just plain ridiculous. My point is that if you move and love how healthy you are given how much you move, don't change a thing. But if you have extra fat that you just can't lose, suffer from repeated injuries, or just lack the energy to get yourself off the couch to exercise because the thought of putting down your Salisbury steak TV dinner is just too painful, then try Approaching the Natural step by step.

Problems exist when we think the solution to stagnancy has to be an "exercise" in the formal sense. In reality, "exercise" can be as simple as walking or running out your door to a friend's house, gardening, taking the stairs instead of the elevator, or commuting on a bike instead of in a car. We don't need gear, special outfits, or a room full of machines to achieve health. Some of those things are fun—trust me, I partake in a few myself, but they are not essential for health. When we're convinced they are, we can tend to take on too much. We get all excited about a new program, class, machine, or regimen, and then wind up burning out a month later and returning to our old, stagnant selves. Just like dieting, initially it can be a fun, exciting, and hopeful undertaking, but chances are, it's not sustainable in the long run. Most of the time we just need to get a little closer to doing what we're designed to do. We can just walk or run right out our door, and we don't even need to put shoes on to do it. Only clothes. Please don't forget your clothes.

Ever seen a garage full of infomercial exercise equipment? Don't overcomplicate things by concocting a big ol' plan with a schedule, equipment, membership fees, and whatever else. I have worked with people who prefer working out at the gym or taking yoga but whose lives don't allow for much time to do either. The end result is that they end up doing neither. I'm all for going to the gym, yoga class, or whatever works for you if you actually do it. If not, start with something simple like a mini-tramp, walks, or jogs because, again, something is better than nothing.

I feel compelled to mention that, for my life at present, the mini-trampoline, or "rebounder," is where it's at. Like walking and running it's a weight-bearing exercise, but highly efficient and extremely low impact. Weight-bearing exercises have been shown to improve both muscle strength and bone health. With each step you push against gravity, and your body compensates by strengthening its own structure. Jumping on a mini-tramp works the same way. In fact, in 1979, NASA found that rebounding didn't inordinately stress out any one part of the body, and applied a nice even impact on every single cell in the body, making it more efficient and easier on the body than both walking and running. Of course humans didn't exactly evolve in a forest of trampolines. We walked and we ran, but for my schedule and life, hitting the trampoline for fifteen minutes a day with a barefoot run thrown in once or twice a week is pretty much all I can muster. I can jump in my living room and keep an eye on the kids at the same time. When my twins hit school age I'll bring back a little more running into my regimen. For now I'm where I can and want to be. Remember, it's "Approaching the Natural," not "Express Elevator to the Natural." However, if at some point you see me walking in the forest in a loincloth, eating wild roots, leaves, and berries, you'll know I've gone all the way, but at the same time you might want to avoid direct eye contact.

While there are plenty of times when a complete change is merited—for example, when facing a life-threatening illness —most of the time just taking little steps starts us on the journey to health. Think of anything you do as a new behavior, and one that gets a little easier to do each time you do it. Then the more you do it the better you start to feel, and perhaps the more steps you'll want to take toward the Natural. You can incorporate the crazier and fun ways to exercise once you've made movement a "normal" part of your life.

Let's pretend you're the guy sitting on the couch with the Salisbury steak, and that the word "stagnant" barely gets at the lack of movement in your life. Here's what I want you to do. Put this book down, walk to the other side of the room, and then back to the book. Sorry you had to go, but rest assured you were missed. For the record, you just moved your body, and I order you to feel pretty darn good about yourself. You may be thinking how ridiculous that little walk was, but what you just did is meaningful in a very real way. You got up and moved. So what if it was just across the room. It was farther than you would've walked otherwise, and by doing so you began a very powerful process of change in your life. Even if you're not presently the pretend stagnant guy, you may still need to begin the process at some point in the future. Little steps will get you started and remind you that something is better than nothing. In fact, "Something Better Than Nothing" could have been the title of this book.

How did your little jaunt across the room feel, truly? Choosing to do something good for yourself, no matter how small, is empowering and over time will play a crucial role in your journey to health and happiness. I'll get into this deeper in Chapter Four, but infusing mindfulness into your actions will help get you there plain and simple.

Walking across the room with health and well-being as your goal is a very different animal from walking across the room to get a Twinkie. When you make mindful, conscious choices for your own good, you eventually become somebody who takes care of herself. You also build self-confidence and self-esteem because by actually taking steps you send yourself the message that you have the power to change your own life. Speaking of Twinkies, I recently read the ingredients on the package for the first time ever—astounding how many things go into the making of those tasty treats. I seem to remember one of the ingredients being motor oil, which would be healthy if you took my "body as car" metaphor literally.

*

As you can see, movement can be as simple as getting up and walking across the room, but let's see how "Approaching the Natural" might apply beyond that. The next step could be walking down the hall. Better yet, follow my eight-year-old daughter's lead—she pretty much skips wherever she needs to go, including down the hall to grab "Lavender Cuckoo," her toy raven. Seriously, when is the last time you skipped? Next, you might take the stairs instead of the elevator just once a week to start. Eventually try it twice a week and so on and so forth. The next step might be adding more walking to your day by parking a little further from your office.

Maybe a few days, weeks, or even months later (whenever you feel ready), try walking slowly for 15 minutes wherever you can. This can be on the ground or a treadmill. Just get up a mere 15 minutes earlier than usual, or finish your day with the walk. If that gets you where you want to go, hold there. If not, take another step by adding a few more minutes, or increasing your speed just a smidge. Even increasing the duration of your walk by a minute is significant and won't force you to rearrange your whole schedule. Increase your time and speed incrementally until you can lightly jog for thirty minutes. If you are doing this on a treadmill, try intermittently increasing the incline and/or speed during your run, making the experience a little more like walking /running on natural terrain. At some point you might move your walk or run outside. You may decide to slip off your shoes for a few minutes. There's a good chance that by now you are feeling a little better in body and mind, and you are thinking, "if I feel this good here, I wonder what'll happen if I ramp it up a bit more?" This may be a good time to try out running. If barefooting is too much too soon, wear the shoes. Whatever it takes to get you going. But you know how to go further if you choose to. Eventually try walking or running some trails, barefoot on the dirt. Don't even get me started on the benefits of electrically grounding your body to the bare earth. Seriously, don't get me started. Just wait until the next chapter.

Here is how you can apply the Approaching the Natural philosophy to weight lifting in case you are a fan. You know all those machines you see at the gym? Well it turns out that more injuries occur on those machines than on free weights. This is because machines isolate muscle groups in a way that is totally and completely unnatural to the human body. According to Lou Schuler and Alwyn Cosgrove, in *The New Rules of Lifting*, "1. Many machines force your joints into unnatural ranges of motion, creating damage that may take years of treatment to repair, 2. Most machines prevent your body from doing the most important and useful muscle-building movements." Picking up something off the ground doesn't use one muscle. The machinery of the human body is intricate and complex. It simply cannot be sufficiently addressed by a machine that exercises a single bicep. Our muscles work together in incredibly complex ways, and healthy strengthening comes from movements that are as close to real life as possible. For instance, lifting free weights or using a Jungle Gym (see the resources page), with correct form and full range of motion, properly engages all the muscle groups for any particular movement.

*

Improving your health doesn't always mean adding something in—more movement, more exercise, more pills, or more food. Approaching the Natural refers to a naturally balanced state, which sometimes means removing or decreasing things a bit. With exercise this could mean reducing the amount or intensity of the exercise, or changing the exercise itself to a more natural one. This might include moving from weight machines to free weights to a Jungle Gym. For those of you who aren't moving at all, this means starting to move even just a little.

I have a tendency to push myself fairly hard, so I have to make a concerted effort to avoid getting myself into the danger zone of too much exercise. Remember my stress fracture? In my brilliance, after I healed from my first running-related injury, I proceeded to hurt my other foot.

The injury wasn't running related—my son fell on it full force—so it wasn't my stupidity that came into play that time. I had already signed up for a half marathon that was scheduled two months later, and I was really concerned that I wouldn't be able to be healed and ready in time. It ended up taking me just shy of the two months to fully recover. So there I was two days before the race, running a light two-miler to make sure my foot was fine, which it was. Oh, except that while on the run I got chased by a dog and cut my leg while jumping over a corral fence, and came home with a bleeding leg. Seriously, I couldn't make this stuff up if I tried. In any case, an intelligent person would not have still run a thirteen-mile race after not running for two months with the exception of a two-mile test run two days before the race. I ran the race. I made it nine miles before my calves completely gave out. I crossed the finish line with a stride so microscopic that it was almost impossible to prove that I was actually moving. I had to have a friend pretty much carry me to the car. Good times.

Since that time I have been much better about finding balance and being careful not to push myself too hard. That race was two years ago. I am back into my running and continue to trampoline on the days I don't run. The minimal impact of the mini-tramp and the barefoot running style has kept me wonderfully injury free and feeling great. I'm where I want to be and the balance I have with my movement is something I look for in all aspects of my life. To exercise to the point of injury is taking your eye off the ball. Remember, one of the goals of the Approaching the Natural philosophy is to achieve health and happiness through movement.

chapter three: connecting to the earth

We are animals. We don't think about it most of the time, but we are. We drive cars, work in offices, cover ourselves with clothing, and put "products" both inside and on our bodies. We pretend we are not part of nature by keeping ourselves separate from anything natural. We spend most of our lives without a forest, lake, trail, or stream on our radars unless we're looking at them on our iPad. But the fact remains that we share this Earth with other species and try as we might to distance ourselves from them and everything else natural, we can't escape the fact that our bodies come from the earth and will ultimately return to the earth when we die.

Not only do we cover our bodies with clothing, shoes, and products (i.e. sunscreen) that block us from nature, we are also in a mad rush to cover up the surface of the earth itself. At times it's almost as if the earth isn't really even there. We put materials like asphalt, concrete, plastic, and paint on top of the soil, plants, rocks, and water that make up the natural surface of the planet. Even when we want to walk on the ground, it is less and less available to us. In the context of our health, this is not a good thing, with the exception of mini-malls: *those things rock*. But our disconnection from the earth has some fairly serious repercussions.

I believe that the design of our species dictates that we are happier and healthier: **1.** the more time we spend connected to the earth; and **2.** the more time we spend in nature. The further away we move from the natural world, the more we are in conflict with who we are as a species. Reconnecting to nature brings our existence more in line with who we are, and is another essential part of the "being healthy" picture. The closer you get to the natural, the better you'll feel. Read on so that you won't think I'm suggesting we all move to an ashram, because I'm not. I'm simply saying that if you're not feeling the best ever, getting back to your roots (or in this case getting back to *the roots*) is one way to bring back some balance to your life. Great things happen to us when we "Approach the Natural."

*

The mere thought of a tree-hugger might make you cringe, unless you are a tree-hugger, in which case, right on. But tree-huggers might have been right all these years, at least about the fact that hugging a tree is a good thing. For the record, I don't think they are right about fashion, but that's a different book altogether. Much of what I'm writing about is meant to appeal to your common sense, in the hope that by the end you are thinking, "My goodness, that makes sense. Perhaps we should send him a gift of some kind." Save your gifts. The common sense I'm appealing to here boils down to the following message: *Being in nature is good for us*. Once you actually get out there, on the bare earth, surrounded by wild plants, hands in the dirt, it feels pretty darn good. Our minds clear, we breathe a little deeper, and we may even take a break from our iPhones (the horror) to appreciate the beauty of our surroundings. Let's face it, there is something "beyond words" when we watch a sunset or stand on a mountaintop. I think it's safe to say that it is just not the same watching these things on a laptop.

Most of us feel calmer and think "I really should do this more often" when we get our lazy butts into the forest for a hike once a year. But why is this? Why does it feel so good when we lie on a beach, swim in an ocean, or garden in the front yard? Certainly on a purely animal level, it is not exactly a stretch to see that "being in nature" is where we belong. Streets, sidewalks, buildings, cars, restaurants, and water parks were not always part of our surroundings. Something truly fascinating happens to our bodies when we physically connect with nature, you know...like when we hug a tree. However, if watching "nature" on television is enough for you, stay right where you are. But I'd be willing to bet it's not enough. Then again, any show with a Kardashian in it is both fulfilling and totally natural, so you be the judge.

*

Our bodies are electric. Perhaps you've seen the film *Frankenstein,* or better yet, you've read the novel, since my unsupported theory is that reading is more natural than watching movies. When Dr. Frankenstein attaches the electrodes to the Creature, it comes to life. Seriously, *Frankenstein* is a must-see documentary. But the truth here is that *electricity animates us*. Tissue and cells carry electrical charges and virtually everything we do involves electrical signals trucking around through our bodies. In addition, right now our bodies are full of free radicals, which are positively *charged* particles.

Because the human body is electric, it is affected by the electrical fields all around created by devices like laptops, cell phones, appliances, and power lines. This can be a source of trouble for our bodies. In the book *Earthing*, authors Clint Ober, Stephen T. Sinatra, MD, and Martin Zucker write "All chemical or biochemical reactions are electrical in nature and so are susceptible to being disturbed by external electric and magnetic fields" (p. 234). What can we do to minimize this potential damage?

To answer this question, it is important to look at both the electricity of the earth and the electricity of the atmosphere. Earth and atmosphere exist together in a beautiful exchange and balance of electrical fields. Lightning is a discharge of electricity, which can both descend from the atmosphere and rise up from the earth. Lightning strikes occur on average about 100 times per second across the globe, and these discharges help maintain an electrical balance between earth and atmosphere. Typically the atmosphere carries a positive charge while the surface of the earth carries a negative charge (during thunderstorms this can be opposite).

If humans lived completely in nature like the wild animals we truly are, we would be simultaneously in physical contact (through our skin) with both the earth and the atmosphere. But here's the rub—mostly we're really only connected to the atmosphere. Why? Because instead of having our bare skin touching the bare earth, we've both covered our feet with non-electrically conductive material like rubber-soled shoes, and covered the earth with synthetic materials like wood flooring, carpet, asphalt, and some types of concrete. These materials are non-conductive because they block the flow of electrons (i.e. electricity) to and from our bodies. By blocking electrical contact with the earth, excess static electricity from the atmosphere can build up in our bodies.

To avoid this we can electrically *ground* to the earth, meaning simply that our bodies are electrically connected to the earth. We can do this by either directly connecting our skin to the ground or by placing conductive material between our skin and the ground. When we are grounded, our bodies are at the same electric potential as the earth—the way we are designed to be.

The surface of the earth is full of electrons necessary for achieving electrical balance. This balance can help protect us from electrical interference in our bodies. Again in *Earthing*, the authors describe it this way:

> "Being grounded means your body's internal organs are shielded from any electrostatic or electromagnetic interference in the atmosphere. This provides for a very quiet electrical 'milieu' inside the body where no external electric or magnetic fields can disrupt the internal functions maintaining homeostasis and health." (p. 235)

In other words, being grounded helps the body maintain balance without damaging interruption and stress (there's that darn blasted word again!).

In the context of electricity, the human body is similar to a house. You know that little three-prong socket on your wall? The bottom hole is the ground plug, which functions as a safety mechanism in case of an electrical surge or buildup of excess static electricity. In both of these cases the system is designed for that surplus of electricity to go —wait for it—into the earth. Typically a wire goes from the grounding socket to a copper pipe that is literally stuck into the earth. In the same way, our bodies need to discharge any excess electrical buildup, or better yet to avoid the buildup in the first place. Grounding our bodies to the earth helps us do both.

*

As I touched on in the previous chapter, chronic stress is the major factor that weakens our immune systems. Chronic stress comes from long-term imbalance related to nutrition, movement, environmental toxins and pollutants, emotional trauma, job stress, excessive sun exposure, disconnection from the Earth, or any combination thereof. The human body has evolved to maximize our chances of survival during times of stress. When that stress becomes chronic, our health is compromised.

Our adrenals are the main glands that help us deal with stress. They create and dispatch hormones that cause physical adaptations, which help us handle whatever is stressing us out at any time. While that all sounds well and good, nowadays, not getting our phone calls returned can stress us out, along with an endless list of other aspects of modern living. Consequently, the adrenal glands and other parts of our bodies that help with stress—like the brain's hypothalamus and the pituitary gland—are over-worked and exhausted. We are simply not able to handle so much stress all the time.

Our stress response is designed to confront fairly short-term events like encountering a bear in the woods. We'd either escape, or we'd be, well… eaten. Either way the stress response is over relatively quickly, but during the response a number of physical changes occur. Blood thickens to deal with potential wounds. Blood pressure increases to quickly supply blood to our limbs. Oxygen and glucose kick over to the muscles to help us fight or flee. Digestion slows down, fat is stored around the midsection and pupils dilate to improve our sight. The immune system goes into overdrive to head off infection in the event of injury (and then remember, is weakened in the long run), and inflammation increases. The relationship between the immune response, inflammation, and positively charged free radicals is of particular interest in the context of the electricity in our bodies.

Free radicals have gotten a bad rap over the last few years. But they can be helpful to destroy things like pathogenic bacteria and viruses, to trigger swelling in cases of acute tissue damage such as sprained ankles, and assist cellular communication and detoxification. In his book *Antioxidants*, Remi Cooper writes, "[Free radicals] help with the constriction of blood vessels by influencing the tone of the tissue lining of the vessels. Free radicals are also important in producing vital hormones and activating certain enzymes" (p. 8). Thanks, free radicals!!! So why the bad rap? Because of the severe damage they can inflict when left unchecked. As Ray Kurzweil in *Fantastic Voyage* writes: "Every cell in your body experiences more than 100,000 free-radical attacks each day" (p. 234). Free radicals can literally oxidize (kind of like rust) the walls of our cells.

Here's the 411 on free radicals. Many free radicals are a by-product of our normal metabolism. The oxygen (O_2) we breathe is combined with the nutrients we consume and our cells process these together to produce energy. As O_2, the two individual oxygen atoms are bound together and share a pair of electrons. The molecule is stable and electrically balanced (equal number of protons and electrons —positive and negative). But after it is used to produce energy, the O2 molecule is separated into individual oxygen atoms. The result of this separation is that each oxygen atom is now missing an electron, and becomes unbalanced and positively charged because each has more protons than electrons. These single oxygen atoms are extremely unstable, and I don't mean emotionally. Each becomes a free radical. Free radicals search around desperately for an electron to make it electrically balanced once again. These free radicals are searching for an electron like they are looking for their soul mate, except that any ol' electron will do, so obviously their standards aren't that high. But free radicals don't just find a lonely electron and offer to buy it a drink. Instead they will steal that electron from a neighboring atom or molecule, which unfortunately turns that one into another free radical. My friend Ryane Snow, naturalist and PhD in chemistry, explained this concept to me by drawing it all out on a cocktail napkin, which is easily as good and reliable as a government-funded study. Sadly, Ryane passed away while I was writing this book. Here's to you, my friend…

Free radicals become a problem when we lack the tools to control them. Left unchecked, the free radicals—which incidentally would make a stellar band name—can cause damage to our cells and healthy tissue. When the immune system gets word that healthy tissue is being damaged, guess what it sends down there to take care of the problem? More free radicals and more damage. According to *The China Study*,

"...*uncontrolled* free radical damage also is part of the processes that give rise to cataracts, to hardening of the arteries, to cancer, to emphysema, to arthritis and many other ailments that become more common with age." (p. 93) [Emphasis added]

In *Earthing*, the authors explain it this way: "[Free radicals] continue attacking and oxidize healthy tissue. The immune system gears switch into overdrive, sending in more white blood cells that produce more free radicals" (p. 60). What they're writing about is inflammation—the body's brilliant response to damage, and only a problem when it becomes chronic.

Best-case scenario is that the free radicals do their jobs and are then neutralized by the body: job well done. Damage is kept to a minimum and our immune systems aren't overtaxed. Worst-case scenario is these little buggers get to keep on rockin' unchecked, and are able to throw the best party ever as if their folks were away on vacation in Tulsa. The question that remains is how to keep free radical damage under control.

Here is where grounding our bodies comes in and why tree-huggers may be so dang smart. Let me be clear right out of the shoot. Grounding is physically connecting to the earth in any way. It can mean literally hugging a tree, but it doesn't have to be. I can't even get my arms completely around most trees and trust me, I've tried. Remember the free flow of electrons to and from our bodies that occurs when we are grounded? These electrons are just what the free radicals are looking for. By touching the earth we allow the electrons on the earth's surface to flow freely in and out of our bodies, restoring our electrical balance. If there's a buildup of electricity in our bodies, it can be discharged into the earth. Our bodies would be in electrical balance if we were in perpetual contact with the earth as we used to be. In *Barefoot Running*, Michael Sandler explains it this way:

> "When you reconnect to the negatively charged electrons on the surface of the earth, the buildup of positively charged free radicals in your body that leads to inflammation is neutralized. Chronic Inflammation has been implicated in all types of serious health issues including diabetes, Alzheimer's, cancer, leukemia, heart disease, and autoimmune disorders such as rheumatoid arthritis, multiple sclerosis, and many others. When research subjects were connected to the earth, medical thermal images showed decreased inflammation in only minutes." (p. 18-19)

Again, avoiding damage to the body means less work the body has to do for repair. Less work means less stress.

In addition to grounding, there is one more tool that helps decrease free radical damage: the antioxidant. In Chapter One I listed antioxidants as one of the micronutrients in food along with vitamins, minerals, and phytochemicals, but I address antioxidants in this chapter because they help keep free radicals in check in much the same way as grounding. As Remi Cooper states in his book *Antioxidants*, "Antioxidants are the body's major defense against free radicals...Antioxidants fight free radicals by neutralizing them—they supply the missing electron and so stabilize the molecule" (p. 12).

Consuming antioxidants helps the body neutralize free radicals. What's interesting is that antioxidants, found primarily in plants, work much the same way in plants as they do in our bodies. In *The China Study*, T. Colin Campbell describes it this way:

> "The site at which photosynthesis takes place is a bit like a nuclear reactor. The electrons zooming around in the plant that are changing the sunlight into chemical energy must be managed very carefully. If they stray from their rightful places in the process, they may create free radicals, which can wreak havoc in the plant...So how does the plant manage these complex reactions and protect against errant electrons and free radicals? It puts up a shield around potentially dangerous reactions that sponges up these highly reactive substances. The shield is made up of antioxidants..." (p. 92-93)

Antioxidants, especially carotenoids and bioflavonoids, also give plants their awesome colors. The groovy thing is that we are designed to be attracted to these colors. Picture yourself walking up to a strawberry bush, flush with big, ripe, juicy, red strawberries. What do you feel like doing? Basically we are drawn to those beautifully colored plants, and when we eat them, the antioxidants that protect the plants from their own free radical damage go on to protect us as well. Interestingly, our attraction to the colors in plants kind of shines a little light on artificial coloring in processed food. Kraft makes their macaroni and cheese super ORANGE (!) for a reason. It looks purty and we're drawn to it. Oh, and it tastes like a party.

Grounding and antioxidants are the key weapons in our fight against free radical damage. So when you combine connecting your skin to the earth with eating antioxidant-rich whole plants, good night Johnny! You're a barefoot walking, antioxidant-eating machine. Good on ya.

The benefits of grounding don't stop at helping our bodies neutralize free radicals. Grounding also connects us to the natural rhythm of the earth. In *Barefoot Running*, Sandler writes about the Schumann Resonance, which is the frequency of the earth (average of 7.83 hertz—peaking at 8 a.m. and 5 p.m.), and not coincidentally, "the same frequency our brains use to survive and thrive. In other words, our vibrations are matched or we vibrate at the same frequency of the earth" (p. 19). Getting barefoot on the ground for extended periods of time can help your body sync to the Schumann Resonance, which in turn can, Sandler writes, "[help] us naturally know when to rise and sleep" (p. 20). This is especially useful when it comes to jet lag, as the natural times to wake and sleep change dramatically as you enter different time zones. In *Earthing*, the authors write that:

> "People who travel great distances have repeatedly reported that grounding for half an hour after arrival significantly reduces, if not completely eliminates, jet lag. This phenomenon is best explained by the body sensing different frequencies from the electrons of the Earth and receiving 'local cues' from these vibrating electrons as to time of day." (p. 239)

Grounding also provides the electrically balanced environment the body needs for it to properly function with minimal stress. In a sense the body becomes normalized and is better able to keep itself regulated. All the major systems in the body even out and simply function better when the body is grounded: the immune system, digestive tract, cardiovascular, etc. All this from hugging a tree? Any chance the whole concept of touching the earth now seems a little less odd? Is it just me or is this stuff mind-blowing?

*

Physically reconnecting to the earth clearly helps put us on the path to health, but what about the psychological benefits of re-onnecting to the earth? Here's where I get all touchy-feely about how it feels to be surrounded by the natural world. Think about how wonderful it feels to walk through a forest. Even in rubber-soled shoes, being in nature calms us down and clears our heads.

There is a profound connection between overall happiness and the amount of time spent in nature. In *Last Child in the Woods: Saving our Children from Nature-Deficit Disorder,* Richard Louv points out how a lack of connection with nature can psychologically affect children and adults. Louv writes that Attention Deficit Hyperactivity Disorder (ADHD) can be improved by getting children into a natural setting:

> "Many children may benefit from medications, but the real disorder is less in the child than it is in the imposed, artificial environment. Viewed from this angle, the society that has disengaged the child from nature is most certainly disordered, if well meaning. *To take nature and natural play away from children may be tantamount to withholding oxygen.*" (p. 109) [Emphasis added]

Throughout his book, Louv cites numerous studies showing increased creativity, better language skills, and even an increase in the ability to fantasize in children who spend time in natural settings rather than man-made playgrounds. This is significant because these improvements come from actually being in natural settings like forests, fields, and beaches, and not just from being outside.

I think it behooves adults and children alike to return to, and re-engage with, nature. I think we can agree that we don't need studies to tell us that venturing into a natural setting helps us reset our clocks. However, accessibility to nature can be difficult for many of us, so that's where the Approaching philosophy comes in.

*

In the craziness of our lives, how do we begin to reconnect to our natural selves? When we're super-stressed, the last thing we think about is taking care of ourselves. Instead of treating our bodies and minds really well when we need the most care, we "deal" with stress by smoking, drinking alcohol, drinking tons of caffeine, taking drugs, and eating light box foods. Nice picture, eh? But even in the busiest, most stressful times of our live, there are ways we can truly help ourselves by "Approaching the Natural."

Let me present a hypothetical situation. Let's say you got yourself that sweet-ass Beemer you've been dreaming of, and a great job selling some sort of crap or trading shares of the companies that make the crap. Let's say you picked up this book because you're overweight, stressed out, addicted to ibuprofen and Pepto Bismol, downing prescription meds for high cholesterol and blood pressure, and you want to see if there's something you can actually do about it but that won't require you to change your entire life. Here are the steps you can take *today*.

While the "best" amount of time for humans to ground or be in nature is 24 hours a day, 7 days a week, that's just not possible given your lifestyle. It's not gonna happen. I know it, you know it. But when you hit the street tomorrow during your lunch break to grab a hot dog (ideally one of those antioxidant-filled ones), try taking a second to sit on a bit of grass and pop off the ol' Cole Haans. Even a second is better than nothing. During a commercial break in the football game, step outside barefoot or hold onto a tree, and extend this for a couple minutes. See how it feels as you discharge the excess electricity that has accumulated in your body. See if you breathe a little slower or feel calmer. You might just sleep a little better that night.

Next step? Eat your lunch in the park with your shoes off the whole time. If you're self-conscious about not wearing shoes, place your hand on the ground or lean against a tree, as long as some of your skin is touching it. Want to go even closer to the natural? Take your coffee breaks outside on the ground. Meet friends and talk about anything and everything, except work. As you'll read in Chapter Five, human-to-human interaction is essential and beneficial to our health and happiness.

If you have the time and want to go further, spend a part of your weekend outside. This can mean your backyard, a park, beach, forest, or wherever. Go camping, take up surfing, or walk on the beach. By the way, surfers are the ultimate grounders, as ocean water is chock full of electrolytes that make it highly conductive. If you're tired, lay on the beach with your skin touching the sand. Try gardening, but do it barefoot or lose the gloves so your hands are actually touching the soil. If you take the kids to the park, take your shoes off. If the weather is too rough for you, or you can't easily get outside, pick up a grounding sheet and use it in your house or office. These work by connecting you directly to the earth through the ground wire in your house (see the references page at the back of the book).

I have incorporated grounding into my everyday life. When my twins were born, and I would get up to change one of them in the middle of the night, I found it really hard to get back to sleep. After putting a grounding sheet on our bed, returning to sleep got much easier. My entire family is barefoot outside as much as possible. I've even got my 74-year-old father on board. He still does some consulting and related a funny story from one of his trips. He had flown into Pittsburgh and gotten in fairly late, so he went directly to his hotel room to sleep. As a retired airline pilot, my father is well acquainted with the effects of jet lag, so he wanted to ground as soon as possible. He got up early the next morning and went outside. The only other people outside the hotel were a group of employees taking a smoke break, and he had to pass them on his way to the side of the building, where he found a patch of bare ground he could stand on. Here was this group of employees having their morning cigarette, watching a 74-year-old man casually walk by them to a small patch of grass, take his shoes off, and stand there barefoot for a few minutes. That's the very definition of commitment.

My point regarding grounding is *do what you can, when you can*. Even if it's one day a week, spend five minutes outside barefoot when you get home from work. That's a great feat (no pun intended). If you're reading this and thinking "I don't even own a Beemer, what steps am I supposed to take?" Remember not to over think this stuff. No matter what you are doing, no matter where you are, connect to the earth whenever and however you can. It's that simple. In fact, put down this book right now, go outside, touch a tree or pop off your shoes for literally five seconds, and come back. I'll wait.

Nice work. Good to see you again so soon. Pretty easy, eh?

PART TWO

APPROACHING THE NATURAL MIND

chapter four: mental nutrition

In section one, "Approaching the Natural Body," I addressed all things physical: nutrition, movement/exercise, and physical connection to the earth. Giving the body the good stuff. Now we're getting into what I call "Mental Nutrition." What feeds the mind? What makes the human mind healthy and happy? What are the little things we can do for our internal selves that will enhance the experience of the very short time we have on earth? I begin this chapter with the individual and then expand to the individual's relationship to family, society, and the world. The discussion here is primarily one of achieving long-term happiness instead of the short-term pleasures many of us are seemingly addicted to.

The Approaching the Natural philosophy as a whole is one of individual empowerment. I'm not one to suggest that you blame your situation on "things outside your control" or rely on the "this is what happens when you get older" excuse. Quite the contrary. My message is to take ownership of your life and your choices. Educate yourself about which foods are truly healthy and start to introduce those foods into your diet. Learn how to move in a balanced and natural way and start moving. Educate yourself about the amazingly healthy effects that come from touching the surface of the earth with your skin, and start grounding whenever you can. Know that improving your health and happiness is both completely in your power and empowering. The more you attempt to take control of your life, the more control you find you have.

When I teach I often get complaints about how hard it is to eat healthy. Even with a basic knowledge of proper nutrition, many people erect psychological barriers to eating healthy. A typical response is, "I'd eat healthier more often, but it's such a pain, and going out to dinner with friends is a nightmare." Many people have convinced themselves that transitioning to a healthy diet is not possible, and that they might as well continue with their unhealthy lifestyle. They say things like: "I'd love to eat healthy, but I just love cheese so much I just can't give it up." In reality it sounds more like, "I love cheese, oh my god I can't imagine giving up cheese, I just love cheese so much, there's no way in hell I can ever give up cheese, triple creamed brie, I just can't imagine my life would be worth living without it." Seriously. Regardless, the underlying message they're telling themselves is that they are powerless.

Embarking on a healthy path can seem daunting. In the moment, it is definitely easier to stay on the couch than to exercise. But when it comes down to a choice between the couch and the trampoline, the question to ask is simple: which one will give you long-term happiness? Think about who you wish to be and paint a picture in your mind of what your life might look like if you were that person. Then, apply the Approaching the Natural philosophy and start taking small steps toward becoming that person. In this instance it might mean only a 30-second jump on the tramp if that is what it takes to get you off the couch. We get stuck when we think there's no middle ground—that you either have to completely turn your life upside down, or do nothing.

Here is the truth: *You* have the power to make changes in your life, and can do so at increments so minute that you might be the only one who knows they are being implemented. A major hurdle I face in my practice is that my clients want results overnight, similar to the effects they expect to get from drugs. We have gotten very used to living in a drug-based world. If we are not feeling well we assume there is a pill to make us feel better—and in the short-term this is often true. The problem with this model is that it is not making us healthier long term, and is sending the message that somehow quick fixes can deliver us sustainable health and happiness. It simply does not work that way. There is no diet, pill, weekend meditation retreat, 21-day exercise plan, or "ab-hero maker" infomercial doodad that will bring you long-term health and happiness (note to self: trademark "ab-hero maker"). Unfortunately, the arduous nature of becoming and staying healthy makes people extremely vulnerable to these quick fix "solutions." We so badly want to improve our lives, but the idea that real transformation takes longer than 21 days turns us off to the notion of doing anything at all. Instead we fall prey to always believing that the next diet or magic pill that comes along will be the one that does the trick. I believe these so-called solutions do not work because they typically focus on either the body or the mind, when real results come from working on both at the same time. There is no getting around the fact that transitioning to true health is a long-term effort.

Caring for the mind is as important and crucial as caring for the body. In fact, one cannot be healthy without the other. Healthy body, healthy mind is a cliché that is right on the money. Speaking of money, it turns out it can in fact buy happiness. Or so I've heard. Well, not really, but I'd like to test the theory myself just once, for crying out loud. In any case, when you neglect your mind or your body (or both), you suffer. A stressed mind weakens the body, and a stressed body weakens the mind. Or perhaps more accurately, a body and/or a mind under stress weakens the human animal as a whole. Eat a diet of primarily light box foods, deprive yourself of a good night's rest, and work a job you can't stand and you'll see the effects a stressed body has on your mental state. You'll be a walking ball of irritability, resentment, and anger. Physical health can affect mood in a considerable way. Even Candida Albicans (yeast infections) and gluten intolerance can alter mental states—depression, anxiety, and more. Likewise bad relationships, crappy jobs, and grueling commutes can land us in bed with an ass-kicking illness if we don't keep our health in check. The good news is that when we take care of our bodies and minds we *feel* better in body and mind. Clean body, clean mind—we cannot separate one from the other.

*

Humans experience happiness in a unique way. Whatever other animals feel on that front—and there does seem to be something beyond simple pleasure and pain for animals —humans have their own thing goin' on (you know, scientifically speaking). The "go to" areas of our lives that deliver us joy and meaning are singular to our species— subjects like art, music, ritual, and spirituality. These speak directly to the distinctly human part of us, and the more we include these experiences in our lives the happier we are. In other words, we can feed our minds with solely human Mental Nutrition and be the better for it. As with physical nutrition, the more concentrated the Mental Nutrition, the healthier the person.

In writing about the natural mind, I thought about the events and experiences that bring meaning beyond the joy of the moment. I'm referring to those times that become the memories that put a smile on our faces and send us off into moments of dreaminess: births, weddings, travelling to other lands, being with close friends, and the like. In thinking about this, I've concluded that whatever those events are for each of us, the quality of each depends on the state of the person experiencing them. What I mean by this is that two different people can experience the same event in completely different ways depending on their own level of happiness. At the end of the day it comes down to who you want to be, and the work you're willing to do to become that person. If you're unfulfilled and unhappy, that will affect the way you see and experience your life. Take steps to make yourself happier, and you could likely find joy and fulfillment in places you couldn't previously.

I also believe everything truly fulfilling in life comes with struggle and hard work. Maintaining a successful marriage? Hard work. Being a successful businessperson? Hard work. Being a successful father/mother/brother/sister/son/daughter? Hard work. Educating yourself? Hard work. But what is the payoff for the hard work? A deeper experience of life and a better chance that you'll find fulfillment and happiness *because you earned it*. Money and a job can be handed to you, but not the stuff that truly matters. Confidence, self-esteem, happiness, and health take time and work. There is no way around it. What is left is to just figure out a way to begin the process. I believe finding a step small enough for each of us to handle is the solution.

When going down the road toward long-term happiness, the struggles along the way are precisely what make true happiness possible. You struggle, you suffer setbacks, but you continue doing what you can when you can because you see things happen in your life that, right about the time you are about to throw in the towel, remind you why you go through the hassle of living the way you do. It's easier to stay in bed and watch television than to walk barefoot for an hour at the park. It's easier to throw a chicken-fried steak TV dinner in the microwave than to prepare a chopped salad. It's easier to date around and keep to shallow relationships with multiple partners than to open yourself and commit yourself fully to another human being in a deep and vulnerable way. In other words, it's easier to avoid struggle. The question is whether or not you're happy taking the easier road.

Now I'm craving chicken-fried steak, which, incidentally, was the only dish in my high-school cafeteria that was available every single day. Every. Single. Day. In answer to the question you may be asking yourself, yes, I went to high school in Texas. But hopefully you got the gist of what I was getting at. There is freedom in knowing that though there is inevitable pain that comes as part of being fully open and engaged in our lives, the pain is far outweighed by the beauty, happiness, fulfillment, and love that are manifest in an overarching presence above the day-to-day struggles. You expose yourself to deeper pain, but at the same time, deeper joy. Big picture stuff.

*

Human beings possess the ability to learn and to adapt. We have an innate curiosity, and when we need to solve a problem or accomplish a task, we are unsurpassed in our ability to figure out a solution. Our awesome capacity to use tools sets us apart from other species, enabling the human animal to be hugely successful. We have an inherent creativity *and* an inherent ability to learn. In this way, I believe the more we learn, the more we create, the more human we become. The truer we are to our species and what sets us apart from other species, the more in balance we become as people.

But we have become thinking animals living in a thoughtless world. We are able to survive without fully utilizing our minds in a natural way. Because of a whole host of factors (job, children, errands, etc.), most of us just do not have the time or energy to use our minds in a way that will deliver us happiness. When and if we have a free moment to ourselves we usually spend that time "connected" or "wired in" to our iPads, phones, or laptops. It is no wonder we think quick fixes are the only solutions. In the short term they at least show us something that looks like improvement. But a life devoid of quality Mental Nutrition results in the same existential conflict that occurs when we stuff light box food in our bodies when our bodies want the exact opposite. This conflict creates profound stress and unhappiness in us. When we work and exist at odds with our nature we pay a high price.

When we foster creativity and educate ourselves, the more curious we become, the more self-aware we become, and the less inclined we are to be beholden to and driven by the animal side of ourselves; the side that tends toward violence, dominance, war, and greed. I believe this explains why studies show rates of violence to be higher among those lacking access to meaningful education. The behaviors associated with reaction, emotion, and mindlessness all tip the scale in favor of short-term satisfaction—we lose perspective and tend to exist solely to satisfy the needs of the moment rather than to exist for our long-term well being. Stealing five bucks—short-term satisfaction. Feeling like stealing five bucks, but not doing it because it is neither who you are nor who you want to be—long-term satisfaction.

For the record, I'm all for checking out once in a while with a fun movie, a beer, or a 21-year-old Balvenie (that's a whisky, by the way, not a woman from Balven). Checking out once in a while is a very different animal from being someone who is "checked out." Sometimes you just need some plain ol' fun, and that's that. Balance definitely applies here. We all need breaks and should take them. But if you're taking a break just to plan your next break while neglecting the things you want to be doing, then it might be time to make a change.

To acknowledge that there are things about your life that you'd love to improve or downright change is not only okay, it is empowering. Perhaps you picked up this book because there's a nagging feeling that there is something more you want out of life—a little pocket of dissatisfaction buried somewhere inside you. Maybe you don't have the energy, intensity, and feeling of "being alive" that you had not long ago but that you remember all too well. The good news is that starting now you can take steps, but to truly transform your life you must first accept that there are no quick fixes. You are the one that has to do the work. If you're cool with that, then pay attention to what follows. It's time to take matters into your own hands.

*

I began this chapter writing about long-term happiness versus short-term highs. Quick fixes are the short-term highs that get us through the periods in our busy lives when we could actually devote some quality time to ourselves but are just too dang tired to do so. I am definitely there myself from time to time. We need to somehow find a way to carve out moments to learn, think, grow, and create. You get home after a long day at work, and you don't exactly feel like busting out the easel or the journal. Instead you flip on the television and the Apple TV and you're all fixed up. Literally—you got your fix. And what better to eat in front of the television than a three-minute TV dinner? Ain't that America. Oh, Mr. Mellencamp, bust me some wisdom. This happens for most of us, and in the blink of an eye, years have gone by and we've missed thousands of opportunities to enrich our lives. To quote the Cougar once more: "Save some time to dream, for the dream might save us all." Thanks, John.

In feeding yourself the best Mental Nutrition, I want to show you where you could go even if you don't want to go all the way. Then at least you know, and can go as close as you want to go based on how you feel and how you want to feel. For example, when it comes to physical nutrition I personally stop at the step just before giving up coffee, you know, 'cause I'm a tad addicted to the roast. At the same time I have given up the dark, black, cup o' wonderfulness when I'm feeling run down or am not sleeping well. Also, day to day, I keep my consumption to a minimum so I can enjoy coffee *and* still be as healthy as I want. I found my balance in this regard. I know Yerba Mate would be a good next step on the road to a caffeine-free existence, but have you ever tasted the stuff? It ain't chicken-fried steak, I'll tell you that much. The point is that my choices come from what I know, not from what I feel like doing in the moment (i.e. drinking coffee). The same applies to most things in life. The more you know the better choices you make.

Don't ever underestimate the power of learning. Knowledge is absolutely essential to our ability to make choices that are truly in our best interest. Without feeding our minds the key Mental Nutrition of education, we swim in fear, worry, cravings, and anxiety, all of which end up weighing heavier on our choices than facts. I find this to be especially true, for example, when the protein subject comes up in my classes (which it inevitably does). My students can listen to the facts, but initially not make a change because they are afraid. They conceptually understand that there's more protein in broccoli than in beef, but the idea of giving up beef for protein is way too scary. I take great pains to present my information as clearly and impartially as possible (I'm not exactly on the Broccoli Council payroll) in hopes that this new knowledge will impart healthier choices.

Knowledge is empowering, and that's a big part of the Approaching philosophy. Read, take classes, attend seminars and retreats, but only as much as you can and want to. I've been reading health books and journal articles for twenty years. I've tried different diets, exercises, and meditations, and have finally honed in on a broad philosophy and approach to living happily. You're reading it right now.

*

Is learning natural to us? The short answer is yes. When we feed our minds with knowledge we are enriched, just as we enrich our bodies with heavy box foods (not with *enriched* wheat flour, by the way). Continue to learn about yourself and the world little by little and you continue to grow as a person. You interact with new knowledge—you form opinions, you share what you've learned with others, and you inevitably stumble on aspects of the world you may not have thought were interesting to you. This Mental Nutrition can come from the likes of university, math tutorials, karate lessons, and meditation classes. It can also include taking time to learn about yourself: asking yourself what you truly want, and who you want to be.

There is plenty of research coming out on the brain's ability to grow and expand throughout life when it is used and challenged, proving that learning is truly nourishing Mental Nutrition. The conventional wisdom of the past, that it was impossible to make new brain cells throughout your life, is just that, in the past. By engaging the brain your memory and intelligence can continue to improve well into old age. Michael J. Gelb and Kelly Howell, in their book *Brain Power*, write that "although some brain cells die as we age, we can generate new cells…people of average intelligence can, with appropriate training, raise their IQ, enhance their memory, and sharpen their intelligence *throughout life*" (p. 5). [Emphasis added]

Once this information on the brain appeared, everyone and their mother became crossword puzzle nutty. Crosswords are plenty fun and challenging, but there are plenty of other ways to engage the brain beyond being able to answer thirty-four down—which, by the way, is "AngelaLansbury." I'm here to lobby for some diversification. Think of it like a variety of whole plants versus kale 24/7, but with Mental Nutrition instead. Below I'll tell you about my top three faves, all of which fall under the rubric of engagement, self-awareness, and learning. Everything below can lead to increased knowledge about *yourself*, which is where it all starts. As I write about each of my Super Three, I'll suggest ways you can incrementally begin feeding yourself the proper Mental Nutrition.

Meditation. I love it. I'm not going to marry it or anything, but I think it is certainly one of the most powerful tools we can use to enhance our lives. Meditation has been shown to be incredibly effective in stress reduction, and to increase awareness and the ability to stay present. Being present in the moment brings with it a feeling of peace and calm. You can learn to feel things—fear, anxiety, anger, jealousy—and not be crippled or controlled by them.

With practice and over time, meditation allows you to quickly flick on the switch of self-awareness. For instance, while you may still occasionally get angry, with a meditation practice you'll learn to be witness to the anger (in effect, watching yourself be angry) instead of being consumed by and acting on it.

Meditation is also one of the most effective tools to use in transitioning to healthy behaviors. I recommend meditation to my nutrition clients as a way to assist them in becoming more mindful of their eating habits. A sense of awareness can help prevent you from getting lost in mindless snacking and overeating. Again, it's like a flick of a switch. There's a moment where you become aware of what you're doing and how you're feeling. Suddenly, you see yourself grabbing the crackers instead of just grabbing the crackers. In that moment it is much easier to make a choice that is truly good for you. You may still crave the crackers, but you can learn to be the person who has the power to walk away. Being in a state of awareness during a meal substantially increases the chances that you will stop eating once you feel full.

Here are some sample steps you can take to incorporate meditation into your life…

Take one deep breath, and then know that in that moment you were present and aware. Now breathe one more time, slowly, and listen to your breath. You know what that is? Meditation. No patchouli required. Transcendental Meditation, Buddhist, Taoist, Mantras, Binaural audio programs, guided meditations, sitting up, lying down— they're all good. Try any and all and you might stumble on one you love. But don't overthink it. Just begin with small increments like this breathing exercise: Breathe in for four seconds, hold for four seconds, breathe out for four seconds, hold for four seconds. Feel good? In 16 seconds you made an improvement over the pre-breathing-exercise you. Good on ya.

Whenever you become aware of what you are doing, take a breath. Look up from this book right now. Take notice of what is around you and take a long, deep breath. In the elevator on the way up to the twelfth floor, take a quick look at your surroundings, and listen to your breathing for a moment. These little steps make you present, and over time will turn into habits. You will find yourself breathing more and more.

When practicing meditation, your mind will wander (trust me, everyone's does no matter how much they try to look and dress like Jesus), and then there will be a moment when you realize your mind was wandering. When that happens, just start breathing again. Not to sound trite, but this ain't brain surgery. It's more effective actually, but like new skills, it takes time and practice.

Another tool some use to meditate is the mantra—a sound, a word, or a phrase that is repeated over and over again. I have three ancient Greek words tattooed on my left arm that carry great meaning for me (you would have to marry me to find out what they are). Sometimes I repeat them during meditation. Choose a word and give it a shot. Like with breathing, when your mind drifts off and you momentarily stop repeating your mantra, just begin again as soon as you realize it, and continue on for as long as you can.

A next step might be to take a meditation class. Meditation is an integral part of many disciplines and practices such as qigong, yoga, and tai chi. Even running and other forms of repetitive exercise can be meditative. In *Thrive Fitness*, Brendan Brazier describes it this way: "Active meditation in the form of running and cycling provides an opportunity for the brain to mull over information it already has, while restricting entry of new information...Active meditation, as it's appropriately called, has many of the same mental benefits offered by traditional meditation" (p. 41). Breathing while you walk or run is meditation and exercise all wrapped up into one healthy package.

Eventually you may find a regular time of day, quantity of time, or type of meditation that really works for you. That might be getting up every morning at 7 and sitting in front of a Buddha statue, or gazing at the setting sun every evening. You also might discover—don't forget, because you took that first step—that meditating before heading out into the world puts you in a really great headspace. Kind of the point, right? There are no rules except to feed your body and mind Mental Nutrition if you want to be healthier and happier.

*

Journaling. While writing in a journal you are in a state of awareness, making it a form of meditation. It is virtually impossible to "drift off" and think about anything other than the words you are putting on the paper. Journaling can be as simple as jotting down random thoughts. It can also be used as a tool to delve heavily into issues and problems. One of the benefits of writing in a journal is that it can facilitate the release of feelings seemingly "stuck" inside you. Seeing dilemmas, confusion, embarrassment, or shame written on a page instead of swirling about in your head provides beneficial perspective and clarity. By journaling you learn new information about yourself, find answers in places you never thought possible, become aware of unhealthy behaviors (and healthy ones, for that matter), and get clear on what you want in your life. All it takes is paper and a pen.

I urge my clients to journal about their food cravings and struggles, and to document what they eat each day. A food journal is incredibly effective in expediting the transition to healthier eating. In *Eat, Drink, and Be Mindful*, Susan Albers, Psy. D, writes "A great way to raise your awareness of your mindless eating is to keep a food diary…Do start this food diary before you try to change any of your behaviors …this gives you the opportunity to establish a baseline, rather like a scientist does when beginning an experiment" (p. 65). By keeping notes of your daily food intake you can discover habits and addictions you never even knew you had. Once you are aware of these behaviors you are immediately in a powerful position to change them.

Let's apply the *Approaching the Natural* philosophy to journaling.

First step: Get some paper and a pen. Does it need to be a Coach leather journal and a Montblanc fountain pen? Not by a long shot. Scratch paper and a #2 pencil work famously. Write one sentence describing how you're feeling at this moment—stressed, calm, sad, happy, nervous. OK, you just journaled. You're Ernest Friggin' Hemingway. (Little-known fact: "The Sun Also Rises" was a journal entry—you heard it here first. Literally.) Remember, just the act of writing about your state of mind makes you aware of your state of mind.

When it feels right, build from there. Try carrying a pad of paper and a pen with you. For now don't even worry about writing anything. If you feel like jotting a thought down at some point, great. If not, don't fret. Just feeling the pad and paper in your pocket will flick on the switch of awareness. You might even take a deep breath in that moment. Chances are at some point you will have some idea or a thought you want to get down. When you feel it, do it. Write about how odd it is to write something down. The moments you take to write, no matter what, are for you and you alone, and will become moments you will cherish and protect. Just introduce the paper and pen into your life and watch what happens. To quote Goethe. "Whatever you can do or dream you can, begin it. Boldness has genius, power and magic in it!"

Next step might be writing for a few minutes once a week. If that does it for you, you're done. If not, try writing for five minutes a day to start building the new behavior into your life. Incidentally, a great time to journal is before stressful situations—big meetings, first dates, performances. While touring I got in the habit of journaling before getting on stage. The practice would clear my mind and help relieve the pre-show jitters.

When my band was at its most active, I read a book called *The Artist's Way* by Julia Cameron. Inspired by the book, I got in the habit of writing three journal pages, without lifting the pen from the paper, as soon as I would get into my studio to write songs. After finishing the pages, I would throw them away. This practice was very cathartic and got the creative juices flowing. Throwing the sheets away was my favorite part. You know, destroying the evidence and such. Amazing how brutally honest you can be when you're 100% sure nobody will read what you've written. The process allowed me to clear my head so that I could begin creating. And speaking of creating...

*

Art. Music, painting, drawing, sculpture, writing, photography, ceramics, performance art, glass blowing, mixed media, you name it. Art is the Mental Nutrition that nourishes us in ways that infuse profound meaning and purpose in our lives. Creativity is a definitive human trait. Our species has crafted art for thousands of years to tell stories, express feelings, inspire change, and create beauty. Ancient caves are still being discovered with walls covered in elaborate art. Life without art would be mighty dull and tragic. Scary to even think about, actually.

Like meditation and journaling, creating art has a way of teaching us about ourselves. Making something beautiful in the world, even if only beautiful to you, can be a healing and cathartic process. My good friend Joan Stanford, a Board Certified Registered Art Therapist, describes it this way: "As children we naturally and regularly use our imaginations; as adults we often disconnect and even disown this part as 'silly.' When we engage in spontaneous play or process-based art-making, we reconnect to our *innate creativity and wisdom*. Expressing ourselves in this way is not only enlivening, empowering and fun, it is also healing. We enter the world of possibilities, 'what if,' which is freeing and great for problem solving."

For me, music is the Mental Nutrient that has fed me the best. Songwriting has enabled me to discover a huge amount about myself, admit things about myself, and work through my own struggles. Fear, love, profound sadness, hopelessness, joy, and beauty—I have channeled these into my music. Art can help all of us deeply connect to who we are both as individuals and as a species.

When creating art for yourself, the quality of the work is not important. Many people do not even try because they think they don't have talent. But when it comes to health and happiness, talent is irrelevant. It is essential to remove the self-imposed pressure of creating something others will think is good. Being free to create without fear of judgment allows you to explore and have fun with all different mediums. Over the years, in addition to songwriting, I've written short stories (decently), screenplays (not bad either), painted (scarily), and drawn (like a two-year -old)—and had a great time doing all of them. Making art is an absolutely uplifting, life-enhancing activity, and over time the work will evolve as you evolve. It's a wonderful thing. The only exception it seems is my drawing ability, which has never ever improved. My three-year-old twins can draw better than I can.

Even surrounding yourself with art can be transformative and healing. Filling your life with art that moves and inspires you can make an enormous difference in your quality of life. My home is full of paintings and drawings (many done by close friends, which adds a whole different level of connection to the work). Going to museums, live music shows, plays, films, poetry readings (as well as reading great works of literature), and listening to records enriches the experience of everyday life, especially when you're doing those things with the intention of improving your life.

What can we do *today* to incorporate art into our lives? For many people the idea of making art is as uncomfortable as meeting somebody named Art, but here are some sample steps you might take to introduce a little creativity into your life.

The first step might be to simply find the nearest piece of art on the wall and really look at it. How does it make you feel? Really take notice of the shading, the colors, the brush strokes, and facial expressions. Try something similar with music. Put on an album and *really listen.* Many people hear music, but few really listen. Can you discern the different instruments? Pay attention to the lyrics. How do you interpret the words? How do the sounds make you feel? Does the song inspire you to write your own? Try disconnecting from everything else while you listen—no e-mailing, texting, talking on the phone, or surfing the net. I still discover new things in songs I've listened to for 10 years. Lyrics can mean different things to me depending on my state of mind when I hear them.

Visit a museum, and take notice of what you like and don't like, what moves you and what doesn't. Just experience it with as little judgment as possible. See if a particular medium tickles your fancy more than another. If you find yourself spending extra time looking at sculptures, take note, or better yet, note it on that handy-dandy pad of paper you've got in your pocket. If you are attracted to drawings and/or paintings, what kind? Oil, acrylic, watercolors, charcoal, crayons? How about the architecture and style of the museum building itself or the layout of the museum posters? Architecture, graphic design—the world of art is vast.

After introducing a variety of art into your life, you might try creating a little yourself. If charcoal drawing seems interesting, for instance, begin with just pencil and paper. It is not an all or nothing proposition, so just give it a shot. Look up at the lamp in the corner and try to recreate it. Drawing that lamp means more than the doodles you do while talking to your Aunt Tammy on the phone, because you've put mindfulness, awareness, and intention behind it. You're powerful because you are choosing to create art as a way to transform your life. Again, it doesn't matter if the work is good or not, and you do not need to spend your entire paycheck on a set of charcoals, art paper, and an easel. My three-year-old twins draw me pictures to put in my office. They'll hand me a pencil scratching of what they claim is a helicopter. Well, guess what? It's a frickin' helicopter, because that is how they see it. They couldn't care less if it's an accurate representation or not. It makes them happy to draw.

After a time, you might step further and set aside some time each week to create. Perhaps that is a good time to go ahead and buy some art supplies and equipment or even sign up for a drawing, painting, sculpture, or music class at the local community college. This could lead to a whole new group of friends and experiences you never even dreamed of. You won't know until you try.

*

Understanding the real connection between Mental Nutrition and happiness is the foundation of your efforts in self and life improvement. Real, lasting health and happiness become the goal that drives your steps along the way. Seeing yourself as a human animal that naturally craves enrichment will hopefully enable you to realize the possibility for change. You can create your own well-being by returning a little bit closer to the truly human parts of you. In the process, you will also likely begin to see how dang far we've drifted away from any semblance of a natural human existence.

The "typical" day of the human living in the modern world—bed to car, car to office, and so on—prohibits us from consuming quality Mental Nutrition. We are burnt out, stressed out, and too friggin' busy to meditate, journal, or write the great American novel, much less a health manifesto. We've got children, parents, loud neighbors, roommates, siblings, and pets, and can't exactly afford the time to meditate on a mountaintop in hopes of becoming so-called "enlightened."

So just "Approach the Natural" little by little, getting as close as it takes to make you happy and healthy. The important thing is taking that very first small step to create a better life for yourself. Once you start you are on your way. Everyone has the time to take steps like those I have described, and none are cost prohibitive. Creating art doesn't mean having to spend a bunch of money. Neither does taking up meditation, journaling, or, for that matter, exercise and eating well. Knowledge and intention are the only currencies you need to buy a good life.

chapter five: the social network

"Part One: Approaching the Natural Body" follows a simple progression: feed your body well, do cool things with it, and connect it to the earth. I lay out a similar plan in this section, but as it pertains to the mind. The previous chapter, Mental Nutrition, tackled feeding your mind well. This chapter is about doing cool things with it. I am referring to surrounding ourselves and sharing our lives with people who inspire, motivate, and support us on our paths, and for whom we do the same. These are the people who can *help* us feed our minds (and bodies) the best nutrition and positively influence how we see ourselves in the world. As the circle expands from us as individuals to include the network of people in our lives, I advocate for greater meaning, substance, and joy in our relationships. I believe fulfilling and supportive relationships are natural to our species, and will help deliver us increasing health and happiness.

I originally titled Chapter 5 "Family," but the fact is our lives are part of a much larger network of people. As a result, I will discuss both family and the broader circles of individuals surrounding us in attempting to get at how we can move toward relationships that bring us joy. But in looking for a more apt chapter title, I needed a term or phrase that accurately describes our social interactions. I began by exploring the history of the human species. Humans are tribal in nature, and those species that we are related to the closest—common chimpanzees and bonobos—still run in close-knit communities. As Jared Diamond writes in *The Third Chimpanzee*: "We are just a third species of chimpanzee, and what's good enough for common and pygmy chimps is good enough for us" (p. 23). Since the genetic distance between chimpanzees and humans is a mere 1.6%, I initially figured "tribe" to be a good title for this chapter.

Then, thinking about it further, "tribe" did not seem like a good fit given how most of us maneuver and interact in today's world. There are a couple of main differences between a tribe and our modern social organization. First, a tribe is dependent on the physical proximity of its members. Clearly this is not the case today, as more and more of us move away from our families, friends, and neighbors when we reach adulthood to start our own families or search for work. Also, the nature of the relationships in a tribe seems more intimate, deeper, and I believe more substantial than many of the relationships of today. In fact, tribes are really more like big, extended families with shared responsibilities, struggles, joys, and common goals. This is very much *unlike* how modern social circles function today.

Taking this into consideration, I believe we are each a point in a "social network" that includes family, friends, lovers, acquaintances, coworkers, and so on. I am using this concept as my chapter title because it captures an accurate picture of the modern human's social organization (and references the website-driven socializing that is becoming more and more rampant). But, between you and me, I really want to use "social network" because Facebook doesn't get sole use of the term just because of the awesome movie about them with the same title. Plus their IPO didn't perform well enough to earn them that right. I said it, I meant it.

*

I will argue in this chapter that while it would be pretty much impossible for most of us to return to a tribal way of life, it is nevertheless worth Approaching a more Natural human social organization if we want to be happier and healthier in the modern world. First, a couple clarifications…

When I refer to "family" I mean the tightest circle of relationships you have, and typically those you have had since childhood. For most of us, this means our blood relations, but I draw no distinction, for instance, between an adopted sibling and a biological sibling. Family can be your great aunt or neighbor, and for some of us, friends assume this role. How your family members are technically related to you is less important than the part they play in your life.

Second, I focus only on adult-to-adult relationships. The nature of parent-to-child relationships is one of a biological and psychological dependency and should be exempt from the kinds of choices that I discuss—e.g., which relationships we decide to include in our lives. The only thing I will say is that as a parent, I try to teach my children the value of healthy relationships in their lives by living the example as much as possible.

*

Within the social network, family typically represents the closest circle of humans around us. This a good place to start when tackling the question of how to move toward a natural social existence. A close family unit is incredibly effective in assisting and supporting us on our path to a better life. This assumes, of course, that our relationships with family members are healthy and positive. Big assumption, I know, for the struggles of living in the modern world often prohibit us from having enough time to maintain these relationships well.

Family members typically know us better than anyone, and they have the ability to profoundly influence our lives whether we like it or not. Just mentioning the word "family" can elicit happiness, anger, sadness, and pretty much every other emotion known to man or woman. Unfortunately (or fortunately, depending on your perspective), this also means family members can be mirrors that show us our true selves. This is a scary notion, but not for me...though, of course not, I mean, it would be really uncomfortable to write that here—in fact my "family mirror" says I'm the fairest of them all! A quick aside: When I was in high school, my mother told me that literally any girl in my school would go out with me (and she believed it). Seriously (probably had something to do with my being 5'3" with glasses). Remembering this story, I think her words represent some of the best that families can bring to our lives—support and encouragement, for example—and that a healthy family life is something for which we should all strive.

As our family relationships transition from what they have always been to what we choose them to be, the same goes for our social network. In other words, as we venture into adulthood, we come to realize that we are not forced to have relationships with parents, siblings, cousins, or friends. If we want, we can choose to break off any relationship that does not add value to our lives, and likewise choose only relationships that are beneficial. This choice is much like the transition we make towards healthier foods. We are gaining the awareness that we have the power to *choose* to be happier and healthier.

The idea that we really can choose the people we want in our social network may be a hard pill to swallow, especially when it comes to family members. Most of us cannot even entertain the notion of cutting off relations with parents, siblings, or spouses. To be clear, I am not advocating abruptly putting an end to relationships that are not working well. Rather, I think there is power in knowing we have choices where previously we may not have realized this as an option. The dependency and obligation that make us feel indelibly linked to many of our relationships can cause undue stress, anger, and resentment. By understanding we are not obligated to anyone we gain strength and the ability to change relationships for the better.

When our relationships are rooted in mutual respect, consideration, and love, they can be great sources of joy and support. Furthermore, these relationships can be just what we need to stay focused on what is truly important to us long-term, and can help prevent us from slipping into old or destructive habits. My approach is to take steps to change the nature of all our relationships to ones based on independence instead of dependence, since relationships are healthiest when the participants are involved because they want to be, not because they think they have to or need to be. Like everything I write about in this book, this change is best approached little by little. In doing so we incrementally become happier, healthier participants in happier, healthier relationships.

*

For many of us, modern living simply gets in the way of having close, meaningful relationships with our entire social network. It is extremely difficult to find quality time to spend with both friends and family. We are busy working or looking for work, raising children, paying bills, and trying to save money for the future (yeah, right). Amidst all this we struggle for a decent social life. At best we manage to check in with family, talk to friends, or see people on weekends to grab dinner. Mostly, we are too busy to maintain meaningful, substantial relationships day to day and we feel it as something missing in our lives. We have moved to a more unnatural social existence.

Without a "tribal" presence in our lives, we are living in ways that conflict with our nature and we are suffering for it. Cell phone, letters, e-mail, texts, and video chats have replaced the physical closeness of family and friends that once constituted everyday, normal human interaction. Ironically we live with the illusion of a tribe by the very technologies that enable the opposite to be true. It is as if, because we invented texting, we think we no longer have to be physically close to the people in our lives. This is eerily similar to our belief that a multivitamin is an acceptable substitution for whole plants. It seems technology is fooling us into believing we can still thrive while living unnaturally.

Because there is a balance to be struck within our social network, what is interesting is that these technologies make it super easy to become too connected, and our lives then swing completely out of balance. How many times have you seen someone obsessively hunched over an iPhone, their thumbs setting speed typing records, texting away with a multitude of people, while—this is my favorite part —sitting next to a "friend" with whom they are supposedly hanging out? People are literally becoming addicted to Facebook. I have a client who, when she is slammed with work, has friends change her Facebook password so that she is unable to log in.

When the scales become tipped in the direction of low-quality, technology-based connectedness, a consequence is that we consume less Mental Nutrition. We spend so much of the day texting, Skyping, or talking on the phone that we give up time we could be devoting to our own mental health (and physical health for that matter). Meditation, journaling, and art are all tools we use to know ourselves and to discover where we are in need of more balance, which includes our social network. Again, the happy person makes the happy friend makes the happy spouse and so on. We suffer when we do not pay attention first and foremost to our own lives.

*

A strong social network is one common denominator when examining the healthiest and longest-living people in the world—a group of people who encourage, comfort, and care for them. This community is a safety net of sorts, and probably a few other metaphors, which I've forgotten because I've been texting as I write this. For these cultures it is truly as much about quantity as it is about quality—a constant presence of support, empathy, and love. Having people with whom to share our lives makes the experience of life so much more meaningful and worth living.

John Robbins, in *Healthy at 100*, investigates the longest-living cultures in the world, and attempts to extrapolate similarities among them. Nutrition and movement factor in heavily, but a strong social network does as well. Robbins writes:

> "Your connections with the significant people in your life—*if they are positive and loving*—can prevent stress-induced illness, greatly contribute to your health and healing, and add many years to your life." (p. 226) [Emphasis added]

Big "if," no? For the implication is that relationships that are not a positive influence in our lives can easily have the exact opposite effect.

Hopefully it doesn't come as too much of a surprise that relationships affect both our physical and psychological states. It is very simple, really. The happier we are, the less stressed we are. The less stressed we are, the stronger our bodies are able to be. Having a strong social network is certainly as strong a tool as any discussed in this book, and well worth the effort to integrate into our lives.

How we spend time with our social network is of utmost importance. Throwing sixteen texts to your best friend about a sale at the Sunglasses Hut doesn't do much by way of infusing meaning and depth into the relationship, much less establishing an effective support system. Unless of course your best friend thinks that the very definition of heaven is a sale at the Sunglasses Hut, in which case, you are a super good friend, and start spreading the news. But all things being equal, taking steps toward improving the *quality* of the time we already spend with our friends and family is most definitely part of the Approaching the Natural picture of a healthy social network.

Robbins addresses this idea when he writes of the Abkhasians and the Vilcabambans, two cultures who enjoy not only longevity, but also health and happiness along the way. He writes:

> "One of the great strengths of both the Abkhasian and Vilcabamban cultures lies in how deeply people are in touch with one another. Not only do they plant and harvest and eat together, but people share with their neighbors the experiences of birth and bereavement, of children marrying and parents dying. In this way, the community is able to take part together in the most joyous and most frightening moments of life. No one has to face them alone." (p. 33)

The concept is very simple. It is not just the closer we step individually to what is natural, but it is also having a social network to share in our experiences and support us along the way. The two cultures above, and the others Robbins writes about—the Hunzans and the Okinawans—all live long and thrive within a strong and vibrant social network (oh, and they primarily eat heavy box foods, move their bodies well into old age, and so on and so forth).

As an aside, the comparatively high rate of success enjoyed by weight-loss and addiction programs such as Weight Watchers, Overeaters Anonymous, and Alcoholics Anonymous is due, in large part, to the tribal nature of these programs. Participants share their issues and experiences, and in doing so realize they are not alone while empathizing with others who are also struggling for control of their lives. With this support system in place, the chance for success substantially increases, and even more so when *combined with the other tools* in this book that move our species toward a more natural and balanced existence. Though if Weight Watchers actually incorporated all these tools into its program, it would have to change its name to "Health and Happiness Watchers" (note to self: trademark "Health and Happiness Watchers"). Approaching the Natural in all aspects of our lives will bring about true and sustainable change.

*

Transforming our social network into something just a little closer to a tribe will yield great benefits. Making a balanced social network the backdrop informing the decisions you make about your place in society will result in positive changes in your life. Remember, you are a human *animal*. Devoting time and energy to improving your family life and family relationships is natural to our species and will yield long-term benefits. In the beginning of this chapter, I asked the question whether family, even a dysfunctional one, is worth fighting for. I believe the answer is "yes," because we are in a more natural state as part of a strong, supportive family and social network. But how do we reintroduce this part of our nature? In making the decision to Approach the Natural social network, what can you do today?

Any step you take is profound if done with mindfulness and a picture in mind of what you want your life to look like. Each step you take toward this picture is essentially a message to yourself that you are worthy of feeling good and being healthy. How far you go is up to you, but remember, in Approaching the Natural, trying to move directly from A to Z increases the chances of failure. You will be jazzed in the short term (like with diets), but less likely to make a real long-lasting transition. Moving in small steps from A to B to C eases you into the process of change. At each stage of progress, you can pause to check in and see how you feel before choosing whether to take another step. This is especially important when it comes to relationships because the steps you take affect other people. Taking very small steps is a way to ease you and everyone in your social network into more healthy interactions. The big picture is to do little things as often as you can in the direction of repairing and/or improving your circles of family and friends.

I need to clarify that as I advocate for taking steps to improve even our dysfunctional relationships, I am not referring to abusive ones—psychological or physical. In situations of abuse you get help and you get help fast—end of story. By dysfunctional relationships I mean those that are not "functioning" as well as they could be and are causing added stress to your life. For example, your sister never calls you back, family meals are a yell-fest, or your great aunt makes biting comments about your lifestyle. I believe there are ways to morph these types of relationships into ones that are more positive.

*

To Approach the Natural social network, we must first look at the relationships in our lives and consider both the influence they have on us, and the amount of time we devote to them. Becoming aware of stressful relationships is much the same as becoming aware of unhealthy habits in general. When we are not happy, we need to find out why. First I will discuss approaching healthy relationships, then approaching balanced quantities of time spent in those relationships.

What are effective ways of becoming aware of relationships that do not serve you well? Meditation and art bring increased self-awareness and open you up to new knowledge about yourself, but I think journaling is the best tool, hands down. Take steps like those described in Chapter Four and direct your writing to examine specific relationships. The practice of throwing the written pages away allows for brutal honesty, and you may find dysfunction where you never thought it existed. Use whatever methods result in increased examination of all relationships within your social network.

So what do you do when you notice that a certain relationship is not a positive presence in your life? Let's say you've taken small steps to make journaling a part of your life, and through your writing you've come to realize that your hypothetical friend Lydia is stressing you out. Lydia makes negative comments about your clothes, your friends, and your job, and she constantly dishes out unsolicited, generally biting criticism. You have never taken much notice, as the criticism has been such a "normal" and constant occurrence.

But with the help of journaling, you are becoming aware that the relationship leaves you feeling worn out and resentful. You remember, because you are Approaching the Natural, that there is balance with everything, and that as an adult nobody is *forcing* you to maintain a relationship with Lydia. In the end you decide to continue to include Lydia in your social network because there are enough things about Lydia you really appreciate—she is thoughtful, and has come through for you in times of need. You just finally realize the relationship needs a bit of a facelift. Where do you go from here?

Try this as a first step toward achieving a supportive, positive relationship. Assess how *you* act in the context of the relationship, because the best way to change Lydia's behavior and the relationship itself is to first change *your own behavior.* How much time do you spend with Lydia? If you find you are talking multiple times per day or seeing each other a lot, you might try decreasing the amount of time you spend with her. Use that time instead to Approach the Natural in other areas of your life. Interact more with people who make you happy. If Lydia asks why you are not spending as much time with her, let her know how you feel. I'm not the "new-agey, touchy-feely kind of chap," but I do believe that clearly and honestly communicating gets the point across more effectively than telling someone everything *they* are doing wrong. You might say something like this: "I'm just spending more time these days working to improve myself. Negative criticism about how I dress or about my job makes me feel bad, and impedes the work and the changes I want to make in my life. I really just need to focus on myself right now." Consider this statement for a moment. Have you insulted Lydia or asked her to change her behavior in any way? Have you said she is a bad person or that she is causing you harm? No. All you've actually described are your own actions, your own feelings. In the process, you have also sent a clear message that *you* are modifying your own behavior by spending less time with her.

You may be amazed at how quickly your hypothetical friend Lydia (who, for the record, is in no way related to my imaginary friend Lydia) changes her own behavior. Remember, she too has a choice (whether she knows it or not) whether she wants to have *you* in *her* life, and she may behave differently to accommodate her choice. Either way, if the relationship continues, it will be because you *both* have chosen to continue it. The result could actually be greater mutual respect and consideration. Lydia will understand that in order to have you in her life, she must treat you well. Remember, the goal here is improving *your* health and happiness, not simply continuing dysfunctional relationships for their own sake.

*

Many of us do not have time enough to devote to even our most healthy and positive relationships. In the craziness of modern life, the often minimal time we devote to being with our friends and family can be the most unnatural parts of us. If you have a great friendship, but only enough time for meaningless texts once every two weeks, then there are small, easy steps you can take to regain some balance.

My social network is certainly lacking when it comes to my friendships. I have great friends, and some who have been a part of my life for as long as I can remember. Though I'm not a youngin', I am not exactly old either. (I'm referring to physical age. Emotionally I am very young. Or is it immature? I try not to think about it.) I actually have friends I have known for over thirty years, but the fact is I don't see or talk to them nearly enough. As you are well aware by now—three-year-old twins—I'm a darn busy bloke. It takes a momentous effort to get my wife and me out the door for anything social. Work, finances, carpools, and everything else we deal with eat the days away with surprising speed. Next thing we know months have gone by without hardly any interactions outside of each other and our children. Sadly, the current relationships I have with most friends are confined to texts and rare Facebook exchanges. This is an area in my own life where I am fairly far from the Natural. I devote more of my time to Mental and Physical Nutrition because I need both to keep me going during my busy life. These days my social life is what falls by the wayside, and I definitely miss it.

My wife and I, considering what we have going on in our lives at present, have pretty much been sticking to ourselves over the last few years with only a few exceptions—some trips with our extended families, and a few dinners out with friends. I am not exaggerating when I say a few—as in less than ten times in the last three years. At the same time, we also see the light at the end of the tunnel, as very soon all three of our children will be in school, which will free up more time during the day to work (we currently work nights so that we can be with the children during the day). At that point we can resume spending more time with family and friends on nights and weekends. The fact is, we know how we would like our social network to look, and we take steps towards that picture—a quick, easy breakfast with friends, having someone over for coffee. Here are some other sample steps...

This is where I sound like a walking contradiction when I say that texting can be a small step toward the Natural. For some of my friendships, texting is literally all I have time for. This, I believe, is better than no communication at all. If texting connects you with a friend you would not interact with otherwise, then it is a viable step. As crazy as it sounds, in this regard you are *texting* with mindfulness and intention. You are acting to improve your health and happiness (note to self: next book title, "Texting for Health"). Try sending texts about things that are important to you or your friend. Send quick messages of support and encouragement.

If at some point you decide to Approach the Natural even more, you can get closer without having to devote any more time—just improve the method of communication. Beyond texting, the next step might be e-mail or, better yet, a letter—handwriting is so much more personal and intimate, no? Try using the time you might spend texting throughout the week to write a more in-depth e-mail or letter. Next step might be a phone conversation. Instead of one conversation every month that lasts for an hour, try talking once a week for fifteen minutes. Any time is better than nothing.

Want to try another step closer to the Natural? Video chatting. How great is it to live in an age where we can video chat? I admit I am still amazed at the Jetson-ness of this technology.

Amazed. In my nutrition practice I work with people all over the country and I always suggest Skype for the initial consultation when meeting in person is not possible. Skyping is not the same as meeting face to face, but it is more personal than a phone call. I have worked with many clients who come to me quite upset about their health. Being able to "see" them, and for them to see me, allows for greater connection, trust, and honesty. There is a deeper and more natural connection to be had by actually looking at the person to whom you are talking. Being able to view facial expressions feeds us more "information" than solely a voice.

Of course, the next step would be to connect with your social network in person as much as you can. This might include dinner with friends or family once a month, meeting your "tribe" for coffee, or taking regular walks with friends. Call a friend and coordinate your grocery shopping trips. Joining friends or family in ways that do not require additional time commitments are easy ways to connect. It is not ideal, but it will improve your life. The important thing is to simply begin the process of getting as close as you can to the natural tribal model.

*

The fact is, we are designed to be physically close to the people in our lives. For millions of years there was simply no other way to communicate than to be able to see, hear, and touch the person with whom we were communicating. Because we naturally thrive within a strong social network, even when we cannot be physically close, we are still happier and healthier the more support and intimacy we are able to have with the individuals in it.

Take steps to make your family and entire social network about connecting, supporting, sharing, motivating, and inspiring. Be the support for the people you love, and take steps to make sure they are that for you. Know that a meaningful social network is yet another, equally significant piece of the health and happiness puzzle, and that having one takes work like everything else that makes our lives truly worth living. Joseph Campbell writes: "Our family is a circle of love and strength. With every birth and every union, the circle grows. Every joy shared adds more love. Every obstacle faced together makes the circle stronger."

chapter six:

approaching the natural takes on the world

In this, the final chapter of this little manifesto, I expand one final time into the world as a whole. Similar to the concept of grounding our bodies to the earth, this chapter addresses the idea of grounding our minds, and applies the Approaching philosophy to getting back, step by step, to acting from within the context of our species as part of the larger world. Because humans do not exist in isolation, how we behave affects the planet and all its inhabitants. I will argue that grounding our minds is not only natural for humans, but that when we act from a grounded state there are long-term, sustainable, and positive effects for our species, the earth, and us individually.

The answer to what it means to be mentally grounded to the earth is found in the way humans use the term "grounded" in everyday life. When we say we are grounded, we convey a sense of being centered, balanced, calm, and even powerful. This feeling is similar to how we might describe someone who is a "grounding" presence in our life—they keep us from "floating" away and losing ourselves in unhealthy behaviors or distractions. Grounding your mind is *figuratively* planting your feet (bare, of course) firmly on the earth and knowing where you stand. I will explain why in this natural state we are profoundly in touch with the breadth of our existence and all beings that exist on this earth, and as a result are better able to care for ourselves. Lastly, I will show what is happening to the earth *today*, given our species' current, spectacularly ungrounded state.

*

When we are mentally grounded we are mindful that we are part of this earth. We are focused, calm, and less distracted by the trappings of the modern world, allowing us to be who we choose to be. In contrast, when *un*grounded, we are easily swept up in the craziness surrounding us and end up "floating" around when it comes to our health and happiness. We jump from plan to plan, system to system, and practitioner to practitioner. Meanwhile virtually every other supposedly "wild" species is living their lives simply, eating well, spending time with their families, and moving around—grounded in every way.

For most of us, just "living" is a momentous task. We are running around like chickens with our heads cut off, at times feeling lonely, panicked, stressed, afraid, and confused. Sometimes we are so busy, we do not even realize that we are unhappy, but we are suffering nevertheless. Learning to ground our minds makes us more aware of both how we would like to live, and what we would like to improve in our lives and in ourselves. Also, as you will see, in this awareness we learn to serve ourselves in ways that have benefits far beyond us individually. Once we are equipped with this knowledge, each of us stands a better chance of achieving whatever goals we may have in our lives. Enter the Approaching philosophy.

*

As I wrote in Chapter Three, *physically* grounding to the earth is simple. Pop your shoes off and stand on the ground. It is the way we evolved, completely natural for our bodies, and puts us in electrical balance with the earth. Likewise, being mentally grounded to the earth is a natural state for our species, and in this state we too are in balance with the rest of the world. The only real difference is that it is not quite as simple as standing barefoot on the dirt, so the question is, how do we do it?

We ground our minds by acting "Holistically Self-Interested." In short, my concept of Holistic Self-Interest takes "looking out for number one" to a whole new level. Holistic Self-Interest involves making choices that benefit the entire human animal, body and mind. This, unfortunately, is not how our species typically acts in modern society, and it is becoming more and more difficult to do so the further we separate ourselves from the Natural. With each step away we lose the ability to benefit the whole of us and instead end up serving only parts of us at a time—body *or* mind, not body *and* mind.

On the surface, each of us being self-interested might seem counterproductive to the success of our species. Some would argue that suffering in the world is the result of people (or corporations, who are obviously people) looking out for themselves. The damage caused by these individuals definitely explains why "self-sacrifice," "altruism," and "selflessness" are held up as virtues—they are the polar opposites of any supposedly self-serving behavior. It turns out there is more to the story, and if we look deeper, a different truth emerges. I believe acting Holistically Self-Interested is a different but beneficial way to serve ourselves, and that those who are *self*-destructive are actually *un*grounded, and far from the natural.

Most of what one might call self-interest in today's world is actually selfishness or greed, and not holistic at all. What is important to understand, however, is that both selfishness and Holistic Self-Interest *are rooted* in the instinct to survive that is shared by all humans. By this I mean that the Holistically Self-Interested person and the selfish person are both self-serving but their actions have very different outcomes. Once the difference between the two concepts is understood, it becomes clear how unnatural and ungrounded selfishness truly is, since acting in this way simply does not make us happy or healthy. Selfish actions do not bring us closer to the Natural.

I will illustrate this with some examples. Consider this scenario: Person A hits the drive thru for a Big Mac, six-piece chicken McNuggets, large fries, and a Coke (literally my standard order in high school) while Person B makes a big mixed-green salad at home, topped off with homemade tahini dressing, some raw cashews, a scoop of quinoa, a sprinkling of raisins, and a good swig of spring water before the meal. In both of these scenarios, these people are out for themselves. Both are acting in ways that bring them pleasure and energy, and that technically continue the survival of their physical bodies (i.e., both meals will be burned for energy). However, only one person is acting in a Holistically Self-Interested way, and hopefully by now you know which one. Here is my conclusion: the difference between Person A and Person B is the "*self*" that is doing the acting. Person A eats solely for the psychological pleasure of the moment (a "high")—for taste at the expense of health. In contrast, Person B is mindful of the quality of his or her mental *and* physical life beyond the ten minutes it takes to eat the McNuggets (with BBQ and hot mustard), and instead eats the salad for long-term health and happiness. Acting in Holistic Self-Interest does not just keep us alive, it makes us *feel* alive.

Here are a few more examples of ungrounded, selfish behaviors: **1.** A business owner focuses only on making as much money as possible. He underpays his employees and completely misses an opportunity to enrich the quality of his own life by creating and building a company where the employees are well paid and happy (and arguably more productive). This is the type of company the owner could feel proud of and *fulfilled* to have built. **2.** A parent is concerned only about her own child's education, and could not care less about how children in other towns and cities are being educated. She fails to realize that the country becomes a better place for her and her family to live the more educated *all* of its citizens are. **3.** A physician refuses to suggest nutritional, herbal, or other alternative healing therapies, fearing his patient might actually make more significant gains elsewhere. The physician may lose out on the joy and fulfillment that comes from simply being part of a person's journey to health, no matter who gets the credit.

In contrast, animals in the wild, living in their natural environment, act in Holistic Self-Interest, similar to Person B in the food example above. For instance, chimpanzees in the wild are not obese, they do not destroy their environment, they do not live isolated from their tribes, and they certainly do not spend hours on end sitting on their butts watching *Chimps Gone Civilized*. Instead, they live in accordance with their natural inclination, which is to act for their own long-term pleasure and survival. In doing so they maintain balance with the earth.

*

Beyond understanding the difference between selfishness and Holistic Self-Interest, it is important to understand why greed and selfishness are so prevalent today. This knowledge enables us to more easily Approach the Natural because we learn to recognize actions and choices that do not serve us. Essentially, selfishness is the direct result of the unnatural environment we have created. As a species we are almost completely disconnected from how we are designed to exist, and this separation keeps our minds and bodies far from the Natural. Looking at it this way, it is no wonder making natural choices is so difficult and rare today. To explain why this is, I will provide an example of how it used to be for our species and compare it to how it is for us today. Because I am hungry I will involve food once again.

We, like chimpanzees (man I could eat a chimp I'm so hungry), are programmed to look for the most efficient energy source possible with the least amount of effort. In the wild this worked smashingly for our ancestors, as it still does for chimps, gorillas, and orangutans (except the ones in zoos). When our old friend Uncle Thak would search for food, he would inevitably find some that was perfectly appropriate for his body—wild plants, roots, and seeds grown in nutrient-rich soil. On the off chance he could not find enough of those, he might catch and eat an animal that ate wild plants grown in that same wonderful soil. The point is, no matter how hard he looked, you can bet he would never find a slice of Wonder Bread.

Today, on the other hand, the greatest amount of energy for the least amount of effort is a Big Mac. It is cheap, fast, and we do not even have to leave the car to get it. The Big Mac, I think we can all agree, ain't exactly a chaga mushroom on the side of a birch tree. Uncle Thak's body was just not designed to find that triple-decker masterpiece at the end of his search (or the plethora of other processed, high-calorie, high-salt, high-fat, high-protein "foods"—whey protein, anyone?). We are not either, though that doesn't stop us from scarfing down fast food with reckless abandon. But the mere existence of unhealthy food puts us is in direct conflict with the drive in us to find the opposite. This also explains why, in addition to these "freak of nature" foods, things like money, television, cell phones, and other modern trappings are supremely tempting to us. They give us a disproportionate and unnatural amount of the very pleasure we are seeking, but the end result is a society full of ungrounded minds.

*

So far I have addressed the difference between selfishness and Holistic Self-Interest, and expressed my ideas on why our species seems to be becoming more selfish. Looking at the world from the perspective of Holistic Self-Interest versus selfishness, we begin to understand that we are all individually accountable for our actions. We may excuse or explain selfish, greedy behavior as the result of the influence of capitalism or money, but the truth lies in the fact that we have become as deficient in Mental Nutrition as we have in physical nutrition. Re-nourishing mind *and* body reminds us how to truly take care of ourselves in sustainable ways. We can still achieve Holistic Self-Interest in spite of this environment we have created around us.

Approaching the Natural grounded mind is taking steps toward becoming a "philo-selfer"—a person who loves himself or herself. Philoselfers always act in Holistic Self-Interest because they act from self-awareness and self-care —not contrary to or in conflict with their long-term happiness. We psychologically connect to the earth when we learn to love and serve the natural self.

Deep within us is the knowledge of how we are meant to live and it feels right when we follow this path. By being philoselfers, we *feel* happier, and we *feel* grounded. The effects of eating heavy box foods, moving our bodies in ways that both strengthen us and alleviate stress, connecting our bodies to the natural rhythms and electricity of the earth, creating, meditating, and journaling all resonate perfectly with us. Doing otherwise is to deny our brilliant design and exist in conflict while causing the profound unhappiness that manifests itself in destructive behaviors. Basically, part of becoming a philoselfer is applying the Approaching the Natural philosophy to all the tools in this book, but this chapter is about first recognizing the need to acknowledge and appeal to the innate drive in each of us to take care of ourselves, our species, and the earth. In doing so we turn selfishness and greed into Holistic Self-Interest step by step. Holistic Self-Interest is essentially the broad stroke encompassing all the paths to real, sustainable health and happiness. Approaching the Natural is, at the end of the day, a philosophy of mindfulness, awareness, and personal strength.

*

Grounding our minds also serves us well because Holistic Self-Interested actions benefit the entire earth, of which we are a part. Better for the earth, better for us, right? On our path to a better life, it is crucial to understand that grounded or not, our actions affect the world. We have the power to be both a positive and negative force, as how we treat ourselves affects everything and everyone with whom we share this planet.

The philoselfer's actions that serve him well also benefit his social network, the human species, and the planet as a whole. Conversely, the selfish person's actions cause harm. As Aristotle writes in *Ethics*:

> "So it is right for the good man to be self-loving, because then he will both be benefited himself by performing fine actions, and also helping others. But it is not right for the bad man, because he will injure both himself and his neighbors by giving way to base feelings. So for the bad man what he ought to do clashes with what he does; but the good man does what he ought to do. For intelligence always chooses what is best for itself, and the good man obeys the guidance of intelligence." (p. 302)

I interpret Aristotle's use of "intelligence" to mean awareness, mindfulness, and being psychologically grounded—to be in a state of mind where the right choice for our happiness is very clear since it comes out of thought and consideration.

He argues that the way to help others is to be a philoselfer, to be "self-loving." We see plenty of examples today of people performing "fine actions" and it is important to recognize that there is nothing self-*less* about these people. Those who fight for change in the world do so because *they* desire a better world. Philoselfers have a picture in mind of a world in which *they* want to live, and they are attempting to make that picture a reality. Incorporating the Approaching the Natural philosophy creates a better world because it embraces and condones the individual choice to be healthy and happy. Why try and alter millions of years of evolution by championing self-*less*-ness when we can work on returning to, and developing, our natural "self" even more?

I strongly believe the instinct and drive to be Holistically Self-Interested still very much exists within us, and if we allow it to flourish our species will once again live in balance with the world around us. But clearly, there is much work to be done. I realize there is something a little off about quoting a movie in a philosophy of health book, but then again, this manifesto ain't your run-of-the-mill book so here we go. In *The Matrix*, Agent Smith says the following:

> "Every mammal on this planet instinctively develops a natural equilibrium with the surrounding environment, but you humans do not. You move to an area and you multiply and multiply until every natural resource is consumed and the only way you can survive is to spread to another area. There is another organism on this planet that follows the same pattern. Do you know what it is? A virus. Human beings are a disease, a cancer of this planet."

Geesh, Agent Smith, pretty harsh. Well, except that you're kinda right. Dang. We are destroying the earth in our currently ungrounded state of consumption, consumption, consumption. Where Agent Smith gets it wrong, though, is that we do not *have* to be "a cancer of this planet." While many of us do behave like viruses, as a species we are still more than capable of acting like mammals. By Approaching the Natural and taking steps to re-ground ourselves, we can achieve a symbiotic relationship with Mother Nature instead of the parasitic one we have with her that is so prevalent today. Mother Nature knows how to keep things rolling, how to keep the scales balanced. It is only in our ungrounded state that we fool ourselves into thinking we can do things better than she. This is exactly the kind of thinking that is causing great harm to the world and its inhabitants.

*

I will wrap up this book by providing an example of what is happening in the world given our systemic failure to act Holistically Self-Interested. But first, I found this particularly relevant quote from Albert Einstein that speaks to why mentally connecting to the earth is not only natural, but worth taking steps toward. He wrote:

> "A human being is a part of a whole, called by us 'universe', a part limited in time and space. He experiences himself, his thoughts and feelings as something separated from the rest...a kind of optical delusion of his consciousness. This delusion is a kind of prison for us, restricting us to our personal desires and to affection for a few persons nearest to us. Our task must be to free ourselves from this prison by widening

our circle of compassion to embrace all living creatures
and the whole of nature in its beauty."

When we do not make the effort to break through the "optical
delusion," our species suffers and the planet suffers. We
are connected to everything whether we know it or not.
Here is what happens when we do not break through the
"optical delusion." The crazy amounts of animal products
we are slamming down our throats (gotta make sure we get
our protein) result in the following:

1. The environment is being destroyed:

"Industrial agriculture relies on natural gas to create
the twelve million tons of nitrogen fertilizer used
annually in the U.S., which represents an energy
equivalent of over 100 million barrels of diesel fuel.
It also requires millions of barrels of petroleum to
manufacture the 1.3 million tons of pesticides used
every year (over eighty percent of which is applied to
the four crops—corn, soybeans, wheat and cotton
—that are the major constituents of livestock feed);
to pump the trillions of gallons of irrigation water
these crops require; to power the farm machinery
that had virtually replaced human labor; to transport
and house billions of animals annually; and to run
the stockyards, slaughter plants, rendering operations,
and refrigerated product transportation systems."
(World Peace Diet, p. 184). [Emphasis added]

2. Millions of people are starving:

"Researchers estimate that 2.5 acres of land can
meet the food energy needs of twenty-two people
eating potatoes, nineteen people eating corn, twenty-
three people eating cabbage, fifteen people eating

wheat, or two people eating chicken or dairy products, and only one person eating beef or eggs. Everyone on earth could be fed easily because we currently grow more than enough grain to feed ten billion people." (World Peace Diet, p. 191)

3. Access to fresh water is dwindling:

"While the purchase of one pound of California lettuce, tomatoes, potatoes, or wheat requires only about 4 gallons of water, the purchase of one pound of California beef requires over 5,200 gallons of water." (World Peace Diet, p. 186)

4. And finally, billions of innocent animals are brutalized and essentially tortured every minute:

"At the slaughterhouses, some of which run twenty-four hours a day, living animals are forced into a line and disassembled…workers are constantly pushed to work much more rapidly than they should, and this causes improper stunning of the animals and increased cruelty and danger because many animals are skinned, scalded and disemboweled while still conscious and struggling." (World Peace Diet, p. 170)

In contrast, the Approaching the Natural philosophy holds that it is no coincidence that the very same (heavy box) foods that are healthiest for our bodies and minds are best for the planet, and the most compassionate to all other species. A grounded, connected existence will deliver health and happiness for all because it is a conflict-free coexistence with the other species that inhabit the earth.

*

The great comic book character Too Much Coffee Man proclaims in *How to Be Happy*: "If only I didn't know that ignorance is bliss, then, maybe, I could be happy." While I greatly respect his love of coffee, I do not agree that ignorance is bliss, because even in ignorance we pay the price for living unnaturally. I believe learning more about ourselves is always the better choice, but we need to be aware that with increased knowledge comes an even greater responsibility. In other words, to live happily we must do more than learn who we are and what we want. We must also take steps to become grounded in the process so that we use what we learn in ways that actually make us happy. If we do not, we run the risk of consciously and intentionally hurting ourselves while knowing better—a profound conflict that will inevitably diminish our quality of life.

I will end with this. In a natural grounded state where we are thoughtful of ourselves and the part we play in the world, it is impossible to cause ourselves harm. "Intelligence always chooses what is best for itself" (*Ethics*, p. 302). Our species does not have to continue on its current destructive path; however, it is simply not possible to help others and the earth *unless we first help ourselves*. What can save us is taking steps to ground that which makes us unique from all other species: *the human mind*. In *Ethics,* Aristotle writes: "We do, however, praise the wise man on the ground of his state of mind; and those states that are praiseworthy we call virtues" (p. 90).

We have the power, strength, creativity, and intelligence to work toward attaining personal health and happiness This fact, and the method to improve our lives, is the

Approaching the Natural philosophy. Take care of yourself and Approach the Natural until you are the person *you* want to be. Godspeed.

references

Phyllis A. Balch, CNC. *Prescription for Nutritional Healing.* (Avery, 2010)

John A. Mcdougall, MD, and Mary McDougall. *The Starch Solution: Eat the foods you love, regain your health, and lose the weight for good!* (Rodale, 2012)

Ray Kurzweil and Terry Grossman. *Fantastic Voyage: Live long enough to live forever.* (Plume, 2005)

John Robbins. *Healthy at 100: The scientifically proven secrets of the world's healthiest and longest-lived peoples.* (Ballantine Books, 2006)

Michael Fossel, MD, PhD, Greta Blackburn, and Dave Woynarowski, MD. *The Immortality Edge: Realize the secrets of your telomeres for a longer, healthier life.* (John Wiley & Sons, 2011)

Jared Diamond. *The Third Chimpanzee: The evolution and future of the human animal.* (Harper Perennial, 1992)

Aristotle. *Ethics.* Translated copy by J. A. K. Thomson. (Penguin Group, 1976)

Joseph Campbell. *Myths to Live By.* (Penguin Group, 1993)

Julia Cameron. *The Artist's Way.* (Tarcher, 2002)

Richard J. Davidson and Sharon Begley. *The Emotional Life of the Brain: How its unique patterns affect the way you think, feel, and live—and how you can change them.* (Hudson Street Press, 2012)

J. Morris Hicks. *Healthy Eating Healthy World: Unleashing the power of plant-based nutrition.* (BenBella Books, 2011)

Louise Tenney. *Candida Albicans.* (Woodland Publishing, 2007)

Joel Fuhrman, MD. *Eat To Live: The revolutionary formula for fast and sustained weight loss.* (Little, Brown and Company, 2003)

Patrick Holford. *The New Optimum Nutrition Bible.* (Crossing Press, 2004)

Neal Barnard, MD. *Breaking the Food Seduction: The hidden reasons behind food cravings—and 7 steps to end them naturally.* (St. Martin's Press, 2003)

J. Krishnamurti. *Meditations.* (Shambala, 2002)

J. Krishnamurti. *Life Ahead: On learning and the search for meaning.* (New World Library, 2005)

Douglas J. Lisle, PhD and Alan Goldhamer, D.C. *The Pleasure Trap: Mastering the hidden force that undermines health & happiness.* (Healthy Living Publications, 2003)

Louise Tenney. *The Immune System: A nutritional approach.* (Woodland Health Books, 1986)

Joel Fuhrman, MD. *Disease-proof Your Child: Feeding kids right.* (St. Martin's Press, 2005)

Michael Sandler with Jessica Lee. *Barefoot Running: How to run light and free by getting in touch with the earth.* (Three Rivers Press, 2010)

T. Colin Campbell, PhD, and Thomas M. Campbell II. *The China Study: The most comprehensive study of nutrition ever conducted and the startling implications for diet, weight loss and long-term health.* (BenBella Books, 2006)

Brendan Brazier. *Thrive Fitness: The vegan-based training program for maximum strength, health, and fitness.* (Da Capo Press, 2009)

Bob Torres. *Making a Killing: The political economy of animal rights.* (AK press, 2007)

resources

One of my main goals with this book is to show how easy it is to begin the process of increasing health and happiness. One thing I find really helps is to answer the question people often ask once they have made the decision to improve their lives, which is: "OK, but seriously, what do I do now?" With that said, below are some resources—I use most of these, and as for the others, I have researched them and can wholeheartedly recommend. The following resources are listed in alphabetical order.

Cellerciser Mini Trampoline
www.cellercise.com

I love this dang trampoline and use it six to seven days a week. As I write about in the book, my life is fairly busy, and this trampoline enables me and my wife to move our bodies and stay in shape no matter what we've got going on any particular day. I leave it set up all the time. I do 15–25 minutes every morning, and in addition will hop on whenever I have a few minutes. My kids jump all the time too—I bought the one with the handle for safety. Incidentally, this is the second mini-tramp I have owned. The first one I bought was a different, much cheaper brand, and it broke within two months. The Cellerciser is extremely well built and is holding up great after two years of daily use by my entire family.

Earthing/Grounding Products

www.earthing.com

Earthing is where you can buy the grounding sheets and grounding pads I write about in Chapter Three.

Jungle Gym Personal Strap Trainer

www.lifelineusa.com

I have not personally used this product. It is similar to the TRX suspension trainer I use (listed below), and less expensive. I have heard great things about it from a personal trainer who uses it for his clients.

Healthforce Nutritionals

www.healthforce.com

I have been using these products for years, but especially the Vitamineral Greens. I recommend them to most of my clients. I typically throw a teaspoon in a liter of water and drink it throughout the day. I also use the greens in the superfood shake my family drinks each day.

Live Superfoods

www.livesuperfoods.com

This company's products are consistently of the highest quality. They feature a huge variety of superfood powders (noni, acai, mangosteen, mesquite), plus cacao, coconut, seaweeds, and much more.

Holosync Meditation
www.centerpointe.com
I have been using this meditation program for over two years and I am really happy with it. It takes one hour a day, but like other meditation practices, the profound stress reduction and increased mindfulness are well worth getting up an hour earlier or going to bed an hour later.

Local Love Catering
www.locallovecatering.com
Chef Barry Jones-Horton and Jen Jones-Horton run this catering company in the Bay Area of California. Barry and I team up for nutrition/cooking classes and have a great time doing it. They cater events and also do meal planning and delivery for private homes. "Love" stands for local, organic, vegan, and eco-friendly. Clever, no?

Monkey Bar Gym
www.monkeybargym.com
This gym emphasizes full-body, real-life movement, plus advocates intelligent nutritional support as part of their approach.

Mountain Rose Herbs
www.mountainroseherbs.com
Super nice folks, and great products. I make a superfood shake for my family every day and most of the ingredients in my recipe come from Mountain Rose—spirulina, chlorella, maca, yacon root, chia seeds, hemp seeds, and more. Their herbs are very high quality and come in powders and whole roots.

Recipes and Cookbooks

www.theppk.com

Isa Chandra Moskowitz's cookbooks are just plain awesome.

www.realfood.com

Ann Gentry is a genius with food. Her cookbooks are fantastic.

www.nourishingmeals.com

A variety of easy, great-tasting, and whole food recipes.

Righteously Raw

www.righteouslyrawchocolate.com

I am compelled to put this in here simply because they have some of the best raw chocolate I've had. Just something my wife and I have once in a while for a treat.

The Stanford Inn by the Sea

www.stanfordinn.com

Ravens Restaurant

www.ravensrestaurant.com

The Stanford Inn is a premiere eco-resort located on the Mendocino Coast of California. I am the Staff Nutritionist and Programs Director of the Inn's Mendocino Center for Living Well, which features Chinese herbals, acupuncture, acupressure, art therapy, qigong, meditation, yoga, and nutrition. In addition, the Inn runs retreats that include classes on nutrition, cooking, gardening (at their own Big River organic nursery) plus mushroom and seaweed foraging walks. Their award-winning Ravens Restaurant is vegan and features some of the most creative cuisine out there. The Stanfords were "green" almost before it was even a color.

Transitioning to Health
www.transitioningtohealth.net

This is my nutritional practice. I work with people all over the country, including private and group classes, teaching school-aged children, and of course private consultations. I also offer daily coaching to help kick-start the Approaching the Natural process.

TrueNorth Health Center
www.healthpromoting.com

This retreat and health center is heavy duty, but its approach is excellent. Fully and professionally staffed, this is a great place to start Approaching the Natural. I researched the pricing and found them surprisingly reasonable considering the high quality of the facility.

TRX Suspension Trainer
www.trxtraining.com

This is the suspension trainer I have been using for over three years. This single piece of equipment, like the Jungle Gym XT above, is so simple but incredibly versatile. The exercises are full-body focused and as challenging as you want to make them. I hang the TRX over my door and do a 25-minute workout, combining TRX exercises with the Cellerciser.

booking

To book Sid Garza-Hillman for television, radio
or a speaking engagement or class,
email booking@transitioningtohealth.net
or call (707) 962-4920.

notes

notes

notes